Ibn Juljul's Generations of Physicians and Sages

AF693092

Handbook of Oriental Studies

HANDBUCH DER ORIENTALISTIK

SECTION ONE

The Near and Middle East

Edited by

Maribel Fierro (*Madrid*)
M. Şükrü Hanioğlu (*Princeton*)
D. Fairchild Ruggles (*University of Illinois*)
Florian Schwarz (*Vienna*)

VOLUME 173

The titles published in this series are listed at *brill.com/ho1*

Ibn Juljul's Generations of Physicians and Sages

Translated from the Arabic with an Introduction and Indices

By

Oliver Kahl

BRILL

LEIDEN | BOSTON

Cover illustration: Ibn Juljul's remark that the existence of an intellectual class depends on the cultivation of learning by governments (*Ṭabaqāt* 116). *Wa-innamā yaẓhar al-ḥukamāʾ bi-ẓuhūr duwal al-mulūk al-ṭālibīn lil-ḥikma*, calligraphy by Nihad Nadam, 2023.

The Library of Congress Cataloging-in-Publication Data is available online at https://catalog.loc.gov
LC record available at https://lccn.loc.gov/2023031785

Typeface for the Latin, Greek, and Cyrillic scripts: "Brill". See and download: brill.com/brill-typeface.

ISSN 0169-9423
ISBN 978-90-04-68222-1 (hardback)
ISBN 978-90-04-68223-8 (e-book)

Copyright 2023 by Koninklijke Brill NV, Leiden, The Netherlands.
Koninklijke Brill NV incorporates the imprints Brill, Brill Nijhoff, Brill Hotei, Brill Schöningh, Brill Fink, Brill mentis, Vandenhoeck & Ruprecht, Böhlau, V&R unipress and Wageningen Academic.
All rights reserved. No part of this publication may be reproduced, translated, stored in a retrieval system, or transmitted in any form or by any means, electronic, mechanical, photocopying, recording or otherwise, without prior written permission from the publisher. Requests for re-use and/or translations must be addressed to Koninklijke Brill NV via brill.com or copyright.com.

This book is printed on acid-free paper and produced in a sustainable manner.

To the amazing Rosa Sheehan

Contents

Preface

I remember that in the autumn of 1985, sitting in the small lecture room of a long since vanished Oriental Institute at Frankfurt University, I waited, together with a dozen other students, for the entry of a famous guest speaker from Barcelona, Juan Vernet, whose *La cultura hispanoárabe en Oriente y Occidente* had been translated into German by a member of our staff and published only the year before. Vernet was a polymath, and his talk, delivered in fluent, slightly old-fashioned German, was a memorable tour de force into the history of Islamic science, and notably its development in Arab Spain—an eye-opener for most of us. Along the way, Vernet repeatedly referred to Ibn Juljul's *Ṭabaqāt al-aṭibbāʾ wa-l-ḥukamāʾ* "Generations of Physicians and Sages", and that was probably the first time I heard of this important book at all. In the decades that followed, and thanks not least to Vernet's wonderful lecture, I became a frequent user, then admirer of the *Ṭabaqāt* and gradually realized, not only the value of this text as a historical source but also its literary beauty. It is therefore with a mixture of satisfaction and regret that I am now releasing a complete English translation of Ibn Juljul's Arabic book—satisfaction because the work is done, regret because it could have been done earlier.

I am indebted most of all to Cristina Álvarez Millán for her kindness and generous sharing of knowledge, material, and time. Many thanks are due to Eloísa Llavero Ruiz for authorizing the University of Granada Library to digitize her unpublished 1979 Spanish translation of Ibn Juljul's *Ṭabaqāt*, and to the aforesaid institution for putting a digital copy freely at my disposal. I am grateful to the editors of HdO for accepting my work in this series; to the anonymous readers for their remarks; to Abdurraouf Oueslati at Brill for his competence and cordiality; and to Sanne Hadfy-Kovács at TAT Zetwerk for the fine typesetting.

O. Kahl

Introduction

1 Background

In 1955, in Cairo, an old Arabic text on the history of medicine and philosophy was published by the Egyptian scholar Fuʾād Sayyid,[1] on the basis of a single manuscript that has remained unique to this day.[2] The work in question, one of the earliest of its kind in Islamic literature, is essentially a biographical dictionary interspersed with numerous anecdotes, and bears the presumably original title *Ṭabaqāt al-aṭibbāʾ wa-l-ḥukamāʾ* "Generations of Physicians and Sages"; it was completed in the year 377/987,[3] in Córdoba, by the Andalusian physician and pharmacist Abū Ayyūb Sulaymān ibn Ḥassān, known (and hereafter referred to) as *Ibn Juljul*. The significance of this work as a historical source for our knowledge of the evolution and development of medicine and philosophy in the Islamic world, and notably in Muslim Spain, cannot be overrated; besides, Ibn Juljul used, for the composition of his work, a number of Latin-into-Arabic translations, of whose very existence we would otherwise not even be aware. Already in 1968, Juan Vernet published a Spanish translation of the last chapter of Ibn Juljul's *Generations*, which deals with "sages and physicians of al-Andalus";[4] and in 1979, Eloísa Llavero Ruiz submitted to the University of Granada a thesis (*Memoria de Licenciatura*) which offers a complete Spanish translation of the work.[5] Despite the pioneering merits and, at least in part, ongoing value of these translations, half a century of research has provided us with an enhanced understanding and a more detailed grasp of many aspects touched upon in Ibn Juljul's book, and a new translation therefore seems justified, if not necessary, on these grounds alone; that it takes the form of English may perhaps help to widen the circle of potential readership. Our new translation is framed by a comprehensive introduction and exhaustive indices, and

1 The system of transliteration used in our book is that of the *Encyclopaedia of Islam* THREE, see bibliography s.n. EI³ and, for the rules, brill.com/fileasset/downloads_products/27684_EI3-Instructions-for-Authors.pdf, 8 f.

2 See bibliography s.n. JulṬab.

3 Dates separated by a slash refer to the Islamic and Christian calendars respectively.

4 See bibliography s.n. VerMA.

5 Llavero Ruiz's thesis remains unpublished but has recently become available online, see bibliography s.n. ŶulGen. Those who cannot read Ibn Juljul's original Arabic may here and there still draw some benefit from comparing Vernet's and Llavero Ruiz's Spanish translations with my own rendition of this difficult source text.

© KONINKLIJKE BRILL NV, LEIDEN, 2023 | DOI:10.1163/9789004682238_002

accompanied by enough explanatory notes to make this intriguing but difficult medieval Arabic document accessible also to non-specialists.

2 Ibn Juljul

2.1 *Life*

The following brief account of the course of Ibn Juljul's life is cumulative, drawing upon all relevant primary sources as well as on certain observations already made in pertinent secondary literature; some extracts from Ibn Juljul's lost 'autobiography'[6] have been retained by at least one Arab biographer.[7] However, the interdependence, repetitiveness and overall terseness of the Arabic sources severely hamper any attempt at reconstructing a satisfying narrative of Ibn Juljul's life, and even the few factual items of information are far from sufficient to bridge the yawning gaps.

Abū Ayyūb Sulaymān ibn Ḥassān, known as Ibn Juljul,[8] was born in Córdoba in the year 332/943–944. At the age of ten, he began to frequent different

6 See the final paragraph of Ibn Juljul's epilogue to his present work on p. 110 below.

7 By far the most informative *primary source* is Ibn al-Abbār (d. 658/1260) who must have had access to Ibn Juljul's 'autobiography' (cf. VerMA 445 f. with GueṬab 49 f.) and in fact quite clearly indicates as much at the end of his biography of the latter's older brother, see AbbTak 4/47 (for Ibn Juljul) and 2/22 (for his brother Muḥammad, apparently also known as 'Ibn Juljul'); note here in particular that Ibn al-Abbār, just like Marwān ibn Janāḥ (d. ca. 429/1038) before him, has retained the correct form of Ibn Juljul's filionym, namely *Abū Ayyūb* (instead of *Abū Dāwūd*), see AbbTak 4/47,2 then JanNMD 1/139 f. with note 1118. Next follows Ibn Abī Uṣaybiʿa (d. 668/1270) who, for his part, is largely concerned with reiterating Ibn Juljul's own, highly interesting account on the reception and sophistication of Dioscorides' *Περὶ ὕλης ἰατρικῆς* in Spain, see IAU 2.2/927–930 (Arabic) = 3.2/1036–1040 (English); other indigenous sources include (in chronological order): IḤRis *apud* MaqqNṬ 2/119, ṢAṬab 81, ḤumJM 197 no. 452, ḌabbBu 285 no. 767, QifTa' 190, MarrDh 2/61 f. no. 152, DhaTI 8/675 f. no. 429, ʿUmMA 9/317 f. no. 107, and ṢafWā 13/293 f. no. 4216. For *secondary literature* (as of 2009) see GarIŶ 163b–164b (with the references given 166b) and ÁlMiIŶ 66b–67b (with the references given 69a), but still compare JulṬab pp. ز—يب; further LongIJ *passim* (2014), with caution.

8 Even though *juljul* is a genuine Arabic word—which denotes "a little bell, consisting of a hollow ball of copper or brass or other metal, perforated, and containing a loose solid ball; [or any] small bell" (LaLex 438a)—Fu'ād Sayyid, the editor of the *Ṭabaqāt*, observes that the epithet *Ibn Juljul* is unique in indigenous onomastic literature, and further considers it to be a transliterated and then completely arabicized form of an originally Latin (or Old Spanish) name given to one of Ibn Juljul's ancestors (JulṬab p. يب, 9–13), making him a *muwallad* or descendant of non-Arab neo-Muslims, cf. on the term ChMuw *passim*; ŶulGen 4,5 f. remarks: "No sabemos nada de los nombres de sus padres y abuelos, pero se cree que eran de origen español". If the latter proposition is valid (and it may well be), a Latin (or Old Spanish) pro-

mosques in and around Córdoba,[9] where he heard *ḥadīth*[10] from two named teachers,[11] together with his older brother Muḥammad, who became a traditionist himself.[12] At the age of fourteen, he took an interest in medicine, the subject at which he excelled and for which he became widely known, finishing his apprenticeship a decade later, at the age of twenty-four. Yet he continued, throughout his formative years, to study *ḥadīth* under the guidance of various religious scholars.[13] He also took Arabic classes from Muḥammad ibn Yaḥyā al-Rabāḥī,[14] with whom he read the book of Sībawayh[15] in the year 358/969, shortly before his teacher's death. Among his companions in those days were the historian and philologist Ibn al-Qūṭiyya[16] and the jurisprudent Sulaymān ibn Ayyūb.[17] Perhaps more significant was his association with the Byzantine monk Nikolaos[18] and the Jewish physician Ḥasdāy Ibn Shaprūṭ,[19] with whom,

---

totype of the name remains difficult to establish and nobody, to my knowledge, has so far suggested a plausible etymology along those lines. The Roman name *Caligula* (or some bastardization thereof) springs to mind, but this is entirely speculative—cf., however, LSDic 270a s.v. *caligula* [only post-classical] "a small military boot" and, by extension, its wearer (i.e. a soldier).

9 AbbTak 4/47,5 explicitly names: the mosque of Abū ʿAlāqa, situated near the so-called 'Iron Gate' (*Bāb al-Ḥadīd*) in the eastern city-wall of Córdoba, cf. LéPrEM 208 note 2,-4f. with 206 (map); the Mezquita; and the mosque of Medina Azara.

10 That is, Muslim tradition(s).

11 AbbTak 4/47,4f.: Abū Bakr Aḥmad ibn al-Fuḍayl al-Dīnawarī and Abū l-Ḥazm Wahb ibn Masarra al-Ḥijārī.

12 AbbTak 2/22,-2: *ʿuniya bi-l-ḥadīth wa-liqāʾ ahlihī.*

13 AbbTak 4/47,6f. explicitly names: Aḥmad ibn Saʿīd al-Ṣadafī al-Muntajīlī, Abū ʿAbdallāh Muḥammad ibn Hilāl, Abū Ibrāhīm Isḥāq ibn Ibrāhīm, and al-Asʿad ibn ʿAbd al-Wārith.

14 A famous grammarian from Córdoba who died in Ramaḍān 358 / August 969, see FarTaʾ 2/93f. no. 1290.

15 Sībawayh (or Sībawayhi), a pioneering grammarian of Persian descent who authored a single, untitled work known only as *Kitāb Sībawayh* "The Book of Sībawayh", which is generally considered to be the founding text of Arabic grammatical science; Sībawayh died, approximately, in the year 180/796 in Iraq, see CarSī *passim.*

16 Abū Bakr Muḥammad ibn ʿUmar *Ibn al-Qūṭiyya* "descendant (lit. 'son') of the Gothic woman", a famous chronicler and grammarian from Seville who later settled in Córdoba, where he died in the year 367/977, see BoViIḲ and MoIQ *passim.*

17 Abū Ayyūb Sulaymān ibn (not *ibn Abī*) Ayyūb *al-Qūṭī* "the Goth", a popular preacher and scholar of (religious) law from Córdoba who died in the year 377/987, see FarTaʾ 1/259f. no. 564.

18 Nikolaos (Arabic *Niqūlā*) 'the monk' (*al-rāhib*) had been dispatched to al-Andalus by the Byzantine co-emperor Romanos II in order to assist with the interpretation of a Greek Dioscorides-codex; Nikolaos arrived in Córdoba in the year 340/951–952 and died there in the early 350s/960s, see Ibn Juljul's own account on the intriguing history of Dioscorides' chef-d'œuvre in Spain *apud* IAU 2.2/928ff. = 3.2/1037–1040; cf. also UllMM 61ff.

19 Ḥasdāy ben Isaac ben Ezra, known as Ibn Shaprūṭ, a physician and court Jew of the

among others, he collaborated on the revision of the Arabic translation of Dioscorides' *Περὶ ὕλης ἰατρικῆς*;[20] this collaboration led Ibn Juljul to the publication of two separate pharmacognostic works[21] and explains his reputation not only as a sagacious physician but also as a skilled pharmacist.[22] At some indeterminate point, probably in his late thirties, he became the personal physician of the caliph Hishām II al-Mu'ayyad bi-llāh, whose long reign began in 366/976. The date of Ibn Juljul's death is not known—however, as Saʿīd ibn Muḥammad Ibn al-Baghūnish of Toledo (born in 369/979) was his medical pupil, Ibn Juljul must have lived at least until about the year 384/994, when Saʿīd would have reached the age of an apprentice.[23] There are no indications that Ibn Juljul ever resided anywhere else than in Córdoba, nor that he ever left al-Andalus.[24]

2.2 *Works*

Ibn Juljul is credited with the composition of the following works:

1. *Ṭabaqāt al-aṭibbā' wa-l-ḥukamā'* "Generations of Physicians and Sages" (completed in 377/987).[25]

Umayyad rulers in Córdoba; he originally came from Jaén and died around the year 359/970, see WaḤSh *passim*.

20 Cf. the source cited in note 18 above.

21 For these see p. 5 below, nos 2 and 3.

22 Cf. IAU 2.2/927 f. = 3.2/1036 f. [13.36.1].

23 Saʿīd ibn Muḥammad Ibn al-Baghūnish had studied mathematics and medicine in Córdoba before returning to his hometown Toledo; the date of his birth is given indirectly by AbbTak 4/81,5 f. who says that Ibn al-Baghūnish died in 444/1052 *aged 75* (*lunar*) *years*. Cf. also JulṬab p. يز, 14–19.

24 Note in passing that Ibn Faḍlallāh al-ʿUmarī (d. 749/1349) gives an isolated, rather fanciful description of Ibn Juljul in rhymed prose; the passage in question surely tells us more about al-ʿUmarī's eloquence and imagination than about Ibn Juljul's life, but it may nonetheless be worth recording:

حكيم فاض بحره التيار، وفات سرى الكواكب ذكره السيار؛ وحام على المجرة ووردها، وجفا بطبه بنات نعش ووأدها؛ ولح على عارض الحرارة وأطفأ موقدها، وحل مجالس الملوك وحل عقدها؛ وخزى به المرض واكتئب، وحصل بصناعته الأموال واكتسب؛ ولم يكن ممن يتهور في إقدام، ولا يتصور أن ينقل إلى ذي سفالة أقدام؛ فكان مدة حياته موقرا، ولا يطأ أخمصه إلا حريرا وعبقرا

"A sage whose ocean swells the lakes, and whose renown the circling planets overtakes; he roams the galaxy and there does thrive, his medicine eclipses the 'daughters of the bier' [constellation *Ursa*] and so he buries them alive; the rise of fever heat he tackles and stifles thoroughly its fire, the kings' assemblies he attends and solves all problems be they dire; he puts disease to shame and turns it into health, and with his skill gains money and wealth; not one to rush headlong into danger, nor to approach some wretched stranger; throughout his life serene he stayed, and in public only wore silk brocade", see ʿUmMA 9/317,17–21.

25 **Ed.** see JulṬab, **tr.** (Spanish) see ŶulGen. **Testes:** AbbTak 4/47 no. 3119,-5 f. ("completed at

2. *Tafsīr asmāʾ al-adwiya al-mufrada min kitāb Diyūsqūrīdas* "Explanation of the Names of Simple Drugs in the Book of Dioscorides" (completed in 372/982).[26]
3. *Maqāla fī Dhikr al-adwiyat allatī lam yadhkurhā Diyūsqūrīdas fī kitābihī* "Treatise on Recounting the Drugs which are not Mentioned by Dioscorides in his Book", also known as *Maqāla thāmina Nadhkuru fīhā mā qaṣṣara Diyūsqūrīdas ʿan dhikrihī fī kitābihī* "An Eighth Treatise wherein we Recount that which Dioscorides Failed to Mention in his Book".[27]
4. *Maqāla fī Adwiyat al-tiryāq* "Treatise on the Components of the Theriac".[28]
5. *Risālat al-Tabyīn fīmā ghalaṭa fīhī baʿḍ al-mutaṭabbibīn* "Epistle on the Clarification of the Errors of Some Physicians" (lost).[29]
6. *Kitāb al-Nabāt* "Book of Plants" (lost; pseudo?).[30]
7. *Kitāb fī l-Istidrāk lil-aghālīṭ fī l-adwiya* "Book on the Correction of Mistakes about Drugs" (lost; pseudo?).[31]

---

the beginning [*fī ṣadr*] of the year 377 [June–July 987]"); QifTaʾ 190,5 ff. refers to the work as *Taʾrīkh al-ḥukamāʾ* "History of Sages" and describes it as a small writing (*taṣnīf ṣaghīr*) "which quenches nobody's thirst [read *ghalīl^an^* instead of *ʿalīl^an^*]—and how else could it be, seeing that (the author) offers so little from among such a vast (pool of information)! He presented (his material) nicely, though"; IAU 2.2/931 no. 4 paraphrases the work's title as "a book that contains some stories about physicians and philosophers" (*kitāb yataḍammanu dhikr shayʾ min akhbār al-aṭibbāʾ wa-l-falāsifa*); ḤumJM 197 no. 452 and ḌabbBu 285,-3 f. speak of "a book offering stories about the physicians of al-Andalus" (*kitāb fī akhbār al-aṭibbāʾ bi-l-Andalus*); DhaTI 8/676,12 calls the work *Taʾrīkh lil-aṭibbāʾ wa-l-falāsifa* "History of Physicians and Philosophers"; further see JulṬab p. ج. Cf. also UllMed 229 f., GaS 3/309 no. 1, DietIDj *passim*, ÁlMiIŶ 68b and GarIŶ 165 no. 5 (with the literature quoted there).

26 **Ed.** and **tr.** see GarLib. **Testis:** IAU 2.2/930 no. 1 ("completed in the month of Rabīʿ al-Ākhir of the year 372 [October 982]"). Cf. also UllMed 268, GaS 3/309 no. 2, DietIDj *passim*, UllMM 62 ff., ÁlMiIŶ 68b and GarIŶ 166 no. 7. The 'book of Dioscorides' is *Περὶ ὕλης ἰατρικῆς*.

27 **Ed.** and **tr.** see DietMM and GarTra². **Testes:** IAU 2.2/931 no. 2; further JulṬab p. كب. Cf. also GaS 3/309 no. 3, DietIDj *passim*, ÁlMiIŶ 68b and GarIŶ 165 no. 3.

28 **Ed.** and **tr.** see GarTra¹. Cf. also UllMed 333, GaS 3/310 no. 4, DietIDj *passim*, ÁlMiIŶ 68b and GarIŶ 164 no. 2.

29 **Testes:** IAU 2.2/931 no. 3; further JulṬab p. كب. Cf. also DietIDj *passim*, ÁlMiIŶ 68b and GarIŶ 166 no. 6.

30 Cf. ÁlMiIŶ 68b and GarIŶ 165 no. 4.

31 Cf. ÁlMiIŶ 68b and GarIŶ 164 no. 1. Note that Sezgin (GaS 3/309 no. 3) registers a work titled *al-Istidrāk ʿalā kitāb al-Ḥashāʾish li-Diyūsqūrīdas* "Correction(s) to the Book of Herbs by Dioscorides" which, in turn, he says may perhaps be identical with the *Maqāla fī Dhikr* … (no. 3 of the above list). In the absence of any textual witnesses, it is impossible to determine the relationship between the two *Istidrāk*-writings, on the one hand, and their potential relationship with the lastnamed *Maqāla*, on the other hand.

8. *Imtizāj al-nufūs* "The Blending of Souls".[32]
9. *De secretis* (< *Fī l-Asrār*?) "On Secrets".[33]

3 "Generations of Physicians and Sages"

3.1 *The Arabic Edition*

The edition of the Arabic text of Ibn Juljul's present work has been established by the Egyptian philologist Fu'ād Sayyid[34] on the basis of a unique manuscript,[35] and published in the year 1955 under the title *Ṭabaqāt al-aṭibbāʾ wa-l-ḥukamāʾ / Les Générations des médecins et des sages*.[36] There is no reason to believe that this manuscript offers anything other than a *complete* repro-

---

32 This presumably spurious work is registered only by Brockelmann (GaL S1/422 no. 16[4]), after a quotation in IQRaw 408,8 (?).

33 A work of this title is ascribed by Albertus Magnus (d. 1280 CE) in his *De mineralibus* to "a certain Gilgil, of Moorish Seville", whom he calls *mechanicus non philosophus* and whose alleged theory, namely that metals are essentially of the same nature as glass, he dismisses as unconvincing and 'stupid', see AMMin[1] III 1.4 = AMMin[2] 163 f. with 284 f. no. 10; cf. also VerIJ 188. It is, however, not clear at all to which (Arabic) writing Albertus refers here, nor whether he had seen a Latin translation of it or merely extracted citations from other authors; equally unclear, of course, is the ultimate source of this attribution, not to mention the actual identity of *Gilgil*.

34 For an obituary see OmFS.

35 Cairo *Dār al-Kutub* (Rawḍat Khayrī) 5636 L [photostat] = GaS 3/309 no. 1: pages 1–75 of a collective volume copied in Rabīʿ al-Thānī 993 / April 1585 by a Tunisian scholar named Muḥammad ibn al-Ẓarīf; the manuscript originally belonged to the Moroccan family (*āl*) of al-Ṣiddīq al-Ghamārī (?), whence it came, in 1950, into the possession of Aḥmad Khayrī of Beheira/Egypt. Other items in the volume include: (II) Yūḥannā ibn Māsawayh's *al-Fuṣūl al-ḥikmiyya wa-l-nawādir al-ṭibbiyya*, pages 76–107 = UllMed 113 and GaS 3/233 no. 1; (III) Ibn al-Jazzār's *Ṭibb al-mashāyikh wa-ḥifẓ ṣiḥḥatihim*, pages 107–158 = UllMed 148 and GaS 3/306 no. 7; (IV) [Ibn al-Jazzār's] *Badal* (*sic*) *al-ʿaqāqīr*, pages 158–166 = UllMed 293 and GaS 3/306 no. 4; (V) Isḥāq ibn ʿImrān's *Risāla fī Tadbīr* (var. *Ḥifẓ*) *al-ṣiḥḥa*, pages 167–173 = UllMed 190 and GaS 3/266 no. 2 ("Nahrungsmittel"?); and (VI) Muḥammad ibn Yūsuf al-Sanūsī's *Risāla fī Faḍl ṣināʿat al-ṭibb*, pages 174–191. For further details see JulṬab pp. مز f. (editor's Arabic introduction). The unique manuscript (formerly Cairo *Dār al-Kutub* 5636 L) is now part of the library of the *Imam Mohammad Ibn Saud Islamic University* (IMSIU) in Riyadh, MS no. 1123.

36 It may not be in vain to signal here that this work-title is somewhat conjectural—it is missing from the base manuscript, and among subsequent indigenous biobibliographical sources only the Andalusian scholar Ibn al-Abbār (d. 658/1260) offers an (almost) clear-cut reference to it, saying that Ibn Juljul "composed a nice book dealing with generations of physicians and sages" (*allafa kitāb*[an] *ḥasan*[an] *fī* [not: *yusammā*!] *ṭabaqāt al-aṭibbāʾ wa-l-ḥukamāʾ*), see AbbTak 4/47,-5 f.; other sources refer to the work in differ-

duction of Ibn Juljul's original, with the notable (and regrettable) exception of some autobiographical remarks which he announces at the very end of his *Epilogue*[37] but which are strangely missing from the one and only manuscript of the *Ṭabaqāt*.[38] Fu'ād Sayyid's handling of this difficult source text is impeccable, by the standards of 1955 as much as by those of today: he prefaced his nicely laid-out edition with a long and thoughtful (Arabic) introduction, put together a perfectly workable critical apparatus, and included in the body of documentation numerous references to indigenous parallel transmissions and relevant secondary literature[39]—the fact that some of the latter is now outdated cannot distract from the high quality and ongoing value of this edition which, over the course of nearly 70 years, has firmly stood the test of time and will have to remain the ultimate point of reference for all future investigations, especially those that are philological in nature,[40] and our present English translation notwithstanding.

3.2 *Sources*

For the composition of his *Generations of Physicians and Sages*, Ibn Juljul relied on a variety of sources which can roughly be divided into written texts and oral transmissions;[41] in most cases, he refers to these sources explicitly, but sometimes an implicit dependence can be inferred. Apart from that, Ibn Juljul

ent terms, or paraphrastically, or not at all, cf. note 25 above and, for further details, JulṬab pp. كب f. no. 5. Eloísa Llavero Ruiz, who of course also noticed this problem, briefly considers the possibility that the copyist of the unique Arabic manuscript 'suppressed' the title, or that his own *Vorlage* already lacked it, but in the end she decides, for reasons not quite clear, that the current work-title is the original one, see ŶulGen 15f.

37 See p. 110 below.

38 Among subsequent Arab biographers of Ibn Juljul only Ibn al-Abbār seems to have been able (or inclined) to draw upon this now lost 'autobiography', cf. Sayyid's observations in JulṬab pp. يج f. Further note that the anecdote which Ibn Abī Uṣaybiʿa (d. 668/1270) transmits in his biography of al-Ḥārith ibn Kalada (IAU 2.1/312f.) on the explicit authority of Ibn Juljul is not found in the extant text of the latter's *Ṭabaqāt*—Sayyid considers the passage, on very good grounds, to be a later addition, cf. JulṬab pp. مب ff.; the same is true for another anecdote which Ibn Khallikān (d. 681/1282), in his biography of Abū Bakr al-Rāzī (IKhWaf 2/79,2–11), allegedly obtained from Ibn Juljul, cf. JulṬab pp. مد f.

39 For a more detailed appraisal of Sayyid's edition see e.g. AnaTA 342–345.

40 Having said that, I did now and then have occasion, in the footnotes which accompany the present translation, to suggest alternative readings or to correct minor mistakes and printing errors.

41 A similar classification is made JulṬab pp. كز—لط = VerMA 450ff.

must also have drawn upon other sources which are no longer palpable. In general terms, he is likely to have had access to Isḥāq ibn Ḥunayn's (d. 298/910) *Taʾrīkh al-aṭibbāʾ* "History of Physicians",[42] even though this proposition is hard to substantiate, given the brevity and radically different character of that writing; likewise, the relatively large number of Greek (especially Galenic and Hippocratic) works which Ibn Juljul was able to cite at least by their titles,[43] suggests a knowledge of Ḥunayn ibn Isḥāq's (d. 260/873 or 264/877) Galen-bibliography.[44] Yet he could not use (and was surely unaware of) Ibn al-Nadīm's (d. 380/990) *al-Fihrist* "The Catalogue",[45] completed only in 377/987, the same year in which Ibn Juljul put a seal on his own work. In those cases where Ibn Juljul cites Greek or Latin authors/texts, he was almost certainly proceeding from Arabic translations—there are no indications that he had any familiarity with either the Greek or the Latin language. Not particularly helpful but no less worth mentioning are broad-brush references to "books of past writers and biographies of those who have gone before us" (*kutub al-māḍiyyīna wa-siyar al-mutaqaddimīna*), "ancient writings" (*kutub qadīma*), "written reports concerning sages of the Greek realm" (*akhbār raʾaytuhā* [!] *li-ḥukamāʾ al-yūnāniyya*),[46] and other such clusters which Ibn Juljul evokes as sources of information in the prologue to his work[47] and throughout; further note an odd quotation from the *Gospel*,[48] occasional references to the *Koran*,[49] to the corpus of early Muslim traditions (*al-athar al-marwī ʿan al-salaf*),[50] or

42 For an edition and translation see RoTA 61–80. Less probable but by no means impossible is that Ibn Juljul possessed copies of Fa/ithyūn's (fl. mid 3rd/9th century) medico-ecclesiastical history, perhaps also titled *Taʾrīkh al-aṭibbāʾ*; Isḥāq ibn ʿAlī al-Ruhāwī's (fl. second half of 3rd/9th century) *Adab al-ṭabīb* "Ethics of the Physician"; or Yūsuf ibn Ibrāhīm Ibn al-Dāya's (d. ca. 265/879) *Akhbār al-aṭibbāʾ* "Information about Physicians"—see for these works UllMed 228 with GaS 3/231 and 263 f.; further RoID *passim*. For some other, rather far-fetched (or chronologically unsuitable) suggestions cf. ŶulGen 2 f.

43 Cf. pp. 134–137 below.

44 For an edition and translation see BergGÜ.

45 For an edition still see NadFih, for a (highly problematic) translation see DoFih. Note in passing that the correct date of Ibn al-Nadīm's death, often given wrongly, has been established already in 1972 by Rudolf Sellheim, see SellIN *passim*.

46 This could be an allusion to pseudo-Ḥunayn ibn Isḥāq's (d. 260/873 or 264/877) now mostly lost *Ādāb/Nawādir al-falāsifa* "Moral Sayings / Precious Maxims of the (Ancient) Philosophers", a genuinely Arabic florilegium which emanated, around the middle of the 3rd/9th century, from the circle of Ḥunayn; see for a detailed discussion of this text ZakPW 1/59–73.

47 Cf. pp. 31 ff. below.

48 Prologue, p. 33 below.

49 Cf. p. 132 below s.v.

50 See e.g. p. 35 below.

to "Greek annals" (*tawārīkh al-yūnāniyyīna*),[51] as well as implicit references to Arabic versions of Greek gnomologia.[52]

Written sources, then, cited explicitly or implicitly, include (in chronological order):[53] Hippocrates *Ὅρκος* **4**, **6** | Galen *Θεραπευτικὴ μέθοδος* **4**, **15**; *Miḥnat al-ṭabīb* **15**; *Ὅτι ὁ ἄριστος ἰατρὸς καὶ φιλόσοφος* **6**; *Περὶ δυσιάτων νοσημάτων* **15**; *Περὶ κράσεως καὶ δυνάμεως τῶν ἁπλῶν φαρμάκων* **7**; *Περὶ συνθέσεως φαρμάκων τῶν κατὰ γένη* **15**; *Πρὸς Γλαύκωνα θεραπευτικά* **4**; *Προτρεπτικὸς ἐπ' ἰατρικήν* **4** | St. Jerome *Chronicum* **P** | Paulus Orosius *Historiae adversus paganos* **P**, **4**, **12** | Isidore of Seville *Origines* (i.q. *Etymologiae*) **15** | Mālik ibn Anas *al-Muwaṭṭa'* (?) **16** | Yūḥannā ibn al-Biṭrīq (*apud* pseudo-Aristotle *Sirr al-asrār*) **23** | Aḥmad ibn Ḥanbal *al-Musnad* (?) **17** | Sābūr ibn Sahl *al-Aqrābādhīn* (?) **41** | al-Kindī *Risāla fī Aghrāḍ kutub Uqlīdis* **14** | Abū Ma'shar *Kitāb al-Ulūf* **P**, **1**, **2** ‖ pseudo-Hippocrates *Ποδαπὸν δεῖ εἶναι τὸν ἰατρόν* (i.q. *Διαθήκη*) **4**, **6** | pseudo-Plato *al-Nawāmīs* **4** | pseudo-Aristotle *Sirr al-asrār* (i.q. *al-Siyāsa fī tadbīr al-riyāsa*) **9**, **23** | pseudo-Galen *Εἰς τὸ Ἱπποκράτους περὶ ὅρκου* **4**. The question of how Ibn Juljul handled these sources will be discussed, inter alia, in the following section (3.3).[54]

Oral sources include (in alphabetical order):[55] Abū 'Abd al-Malik al-Thaqafī **53** (intra); Abū l-Aṣbagh Ibn Ḥayyawayh **42** (intra); Abū Muḥammad Ibn al-A'mā **47** (intra); Aḥmad ibn Yūnus al-Ḥarrānī **29** (intra), **30** (intra), **55/56** (intra); Muḥammad ibn 'Umar Ibn al-Qūṭiyya **19** (intra); Sulaymān ibn Ayyūb **46** (intra); and Yaḥyā ibn Mālik al-'Āyidī **46** (intra). Finally, there is a semi-explicit reference to "the vizier of al-Ḥakam al-Mustanṣir bi-llāh" (**24** [intra]), whom Ibn Juljul cites as an oral informant for a story involving Ḥunayn ibn Isḥāq, and who may be identical with Ja'far ibn 'Uthmān al-

---

51 See e.g. p. 50 below.

52 See e.g. pp. 44 and 51 f. below with notes 71, 110, 112, 114 and 115.

53 Bold numbers in the following list(s) refer to *biographical entries*, as they appear in Fu'ād Sayyid's Arabic edition and, correspondingly, in our English translation of Ibn Juljul's text; the letter **P** refers to his *Prologue*.

54 See notably pp. 15–20 below.

55 This list only contains such Andalusian contemporaries of Ibn Juljul whom he cites *explicitly*. In theory, all individuals biographed in entries **45–57** qualify as potential informants. Consider here in particular 'Umar ibn Burayq (**47**) who had studied in Kairouan under Ibn al-Jazzār and may have provided Ibn Juljul with valuable information about the 'eighth generation' (sages of the Maghreb, **32–34**)—this 'Umar is, in fact, very likely identical with the anonymous trusted person on whose first-hand authority Ibn Juljul relates a story featuring the aforesaid Ibn al-Jazzār (**34** [intra]); and Muḥammad ibn 'Abdūn (**57**) who had travelled to Iraq and Egypt, and may have shared with Ibn Juljul some of his knowledge about the Islamic East. Another "reliable source" (*thiqa*), not identifiable, is cited in entry **43**.

Muṣḥafī (d. 372/982); and there is mention of a handwritten note (37 [intra]) which Ibn Juljul must have been shown by al-Ḥakam's secretary Abū l-Aṣbagh al-Rāzī (d. 379/989).

3.3 *Discussion*

In this section, we will discuss all salient features of Ibn Juljul's *Generations of Physicians and Sages*—the work's formal structure, literary genre, handling of sources, selective character, compositional intention, residual impact, historical substance, and epistemological value.

3.3.1 Formal Structure

Framed by a short prologue and epilogue, the informational content of the text is arranged chronologically according to "generations" (*ṭabaqāt*) of biographed individuals, most of whose activities unfolded, broadly speaking, in the realms of medicine and/or philosophy. There are nine 'generational' chapters of greatly varying lengths, containing a total of fifty-seven biographies of equally uneven scope:

Generation	Biography	Individual
1	1	Hermes I
	2	Hermes II
	3	Hermes III
	4	Asclepius
	5	Apollon
2	6	Hippocrates
	7	Dioscorides
	8	Plato
	9	Aristotle
	10	Socrates
	11	Democritus
3[56]	12	Ptolemy
	13	Cato
	14	Euclid
4	15	Galen

56 In a short preamble to this chapter, Ibn Juljul also names Andromachus, Magnus of Emesa, Diocles and Paulus (Aegineta), but does not honour them with biographies, cf. p. 53 below.

(*cont.*)

Generation	Biography	Individual
5[57]	–	'Alexandrians'
6	16	al-Ḥārith ibn Kalada
	17	Ibn Abī Rimtha
	18	Ibn Abjar
	19	Māsarjawayh
7	20	Bukhtīshūʿ
	21	Jibrīl ibn Bukhtīshūʿ
	22	Yūḥannā ibn Māsawayh
	23	Yūḥannā ibn al-Biṭrīq
	24	Ḥunayn ibn Isḥāq
	25	Abū Yūsuf al-Kindī
	26	Thābit ibn Qurra
	27	Qusṭā ibn Lūqā
	28	Abū Bakr al-Rāzī
	29	Thābit ibn Sinān
	30	Ibn Waṣīf
	31	Nasṭās
8	32	Isḥāq ibn ʿImrān
	33	Isḥāq ibn Sulaymān
	34	Ibn al-Jazzār
9	35	Ḥamdīn ibn Ubbā
	36	Jawād
	37	Yūnus al-Ḥarrānī
	38	Khālid ibn Yazīd
	39	Ibn Malūka
	40	Isḥāq
	41	ʿImrān ibn Abī ʿUmar
	42	Muḥammad ibn Fatḥ Ṭumlūn
	43	Yaḥyā ibn Isḥāq
	44	Sulaymān Ibn Bāj
	45	Ibn Umm al-Banīn
	46	Saʿīd Ibn ʿAbd Rabbihī

57 This chapter only consists of a short account on 'Alexandrian sages', from among whom Ibn Juljul singles out a certain Anqīlāwus, mentioning two of his alleged literary contributions but not dedicating to him a separate biography, cf. pp. 63 f. below.

(*cont.*)

Generation	Biography	Individual
	47	ʿUmar ibn Burayq
	48	Aṣbagh ibn Yaḥyā
	49	Muḥammad ibn Tamlīkh
	50	Abū l-Walīd al-Kattānī
	51	Aḥmad Ibn Ḥafṣūn
	52	Aḥmad ibn Jābir
	53	Abū ʿAbd al-Malik al-Thaqafī
	54	Hārūn al-Ushūnī
	55	Aḥmad ibn Yūnus
	56	ʿUmar ibn Yūnus
	57	Muḥammad ibn ʿAbdūn[58]

Putting aside the question of authorial choices, to which we will return later,[59] the ascending timeline that Ibn Juljul himself insinuates at the beginning of his prologue can be synchronized roughly with our current reckoning as follows: 1 (1–5) prehistoric/mythical; 2–3 (6–14) BCE;[60] and 4–9 (15–57) CE [*Anno Hijra* from 16]. In terms of ethnico-geographical provenance, the biographed individuals can be classified as follows: Eastern and/or Greek 1–5, Greek 6–15, 'Alexandrians' ch. 5, Eastern Islamic 16–31, Maghrebinian 32–34, and Andalusian 35–57; quantitatively, the last category makes up 40 % of the total work.

Regarding Ibn Juljul's own conceptual definitions of the nine 'generational' chapters, they are phrased, in the form of subheadings, as follows:[61]

58 For full versions of the *Arabic* names cited in biographies 16–57 see pp. 124–129 below s.vv. Note that most of the *Andalusian* scholars (biographed in 'generation nine') are only and/or primarily known through Ibn Juljul's accounts.

59 See pp. 20 ff. below.

60 Note that Dioscorides (7) should have been dealt with by Ibn Juljul under generation four; further, that Ptolemy (12) the pharaoh (BCE) is partly confused with Ptolemy the scientist (CE); and that Cato (13) cannot be identified with certainty, and hence his given chronological placement must be taken, for now, at face value. Other, less glaring discrepancies are signalled throughout in the footnotes to our translation of the text. It goes without saying that, as a general rule, the more remote the time, the shakier the chronology.

61 Some of these subheadings, unsurprisingly, also belie (or blur) chronological and, at least

Chapter	English	Arabic
1	those who spoke about medical wisdom and celestial philosophy	*man takallama fī l-ḥikma al-ṭibbiyya wa-l-falsafa al-ʿulwiyya*
2	ancient Greek sages who spoke about and excelled at medicine and philosophy	*[al-ṭabaqa] al-ḥikmiyya al-rūmiyya al-yūnāniyya mimman takallama fī l-ṭibb wa-l-falsafa wa-baraʿa fī dhālika*
3	Greek sages who lived in the (Hellenistic) realm after the (ancient) Persians, and who were renowned in (the fields of) medicine and philosophy	*ḥukamāʾ al-yūnāniyya lladhīna kānū fī dawlatihim baʿd al-furs mimman shuhira fī l-ṭibb wa-l-falsafa*
4	Greek sages who spoke during the Imperial Era, after the founding of Rome	*ḥukamāʾ al-yūnāniyya mimman takallama fī l-dawla al-qayṣariyya baʿd bunyān rūmā*
5	Alexandrian sages	*al-ḥukamāʾ al-iskandarāniyyīn* [*sic*]
6	those who were not of Greco-Roman, nor Syrian, nor Persian descent	*man lam yakun fī aṣlihī rūmiyy^{an} wa-lā suryāniyy^{an} wa-lā fārisiyy^{an}*
7	sages of the Islamic Era who excelled at medicine and philosophy—some of them Muslims, some Christians	*ḥukamāʾ al-islām mimman baraʿa fī l-ṭibb wa-l-falsafa minhum aslām*[62] *wa-masīḥiyyūna*
8	sages of the Islamic Era who lived in the Maghreb	*ḥukamāʾ al-islām mimman sakana l-maghrib*
9	sages and physicians of al-Andalus	*[al-ṭabaqa] al-andalusiyya al-ḥikmiyya minhum wa-l-ṭibbiyya*

3.3.2 Literary Genre

Ibn Juljul's *Ṭabaqāt al-aṭibbāʾ wa-l-ḥukamāʾ* "Generations of Physicians and Sages" is a work that can generally be described as belonging to the medieval Arabic genre of biographical literature, which itself constitutes an old and

in one case (19), ethno-religious realities. Note in passing that the term "sages" (*ḥukamāʾ*) in the title of the work seems to refer mainly to entries 1–14, whereas the term "physicians" (*aṭibbāʾ*) appears to apply more specifically to entries 15–57.

62 Cf. p. 69 below, note 243.

integral part, if not primary expressive form, of Muslim genealogy, traditionist criticism (*ḥadīth*), historiography and, to some extent, belles-lettres (*adab*). Already the genre's earliest manifestations invariably feature, as an important titular marker, the term *ṭabaqāt* (lit. "layers"),[63] which connotes, in the words of Franz Rosenthal, "people belonging to one layer or class in the chronological succession of generations".[64] The significance of the *ṭabaqāt* genre as a mine of source material for our understanding of virtually all aspects of early Islamic history (and historiography) is unquestionable. Returning to Ibn Juljul's *Generations*, it has been observed that the literary form of generational classification enjoyed a certain popularity in contemporary Muslim Spain,[65] but it is also true that it was he who applied this type of writing for the first time, and not just in al-Andalus, to the *history of medicine*.[66] Closely

63 Cf. GiṬab *passim*.

64 RoHMH 82,-4 f. It may not be in vain to cite here some of Rosenthal's subsequent observations on the genre: "The *ṭabaqât* division is genuinely Islamic. It would seem to be the oldest chronological division which presented itself to Muslim historical thinking. It is in no way genetically related to the synchronistic method which was common in Greek biographical tradition and which, at some later date, entered Arabic literature together with Greek biography. It also has no bearing upon the origin of the *ṭabaqât* division that the word was early applied to the four successive Persian dynasties. The *ṭabaqât* division was the natural consequence of the concept of the 'Men around Muḥammad', the 'Followers', etc., which, in conjunction with the *isnâd* criticism of the science of traditions, developed in the early second century of the Hijrah. A marked similarity of this concept with Jewish tradition may be explained as a parallel Semitic development rather than as the result of Jewish influence upon Islam, though the latter possibility is not excluded. The connection of the *ṭabaqât* division with the science of traditions is confirmed by its almost exclusive use in biography", see ibid. 83.

65 Thus, Marie-Geneviève Guesdon says: "Les *Ṭabaqāt* [d'Ibn Ǧulǧul] sont écrites dans un moment où ce genre florit en Andalus: Ḫālid ibn Saʿd (mort en 352/963) avait écrit pour al-Ḥakam II un *Kitāb riǧāl al-Andalus* concernant les traditionnistes, Muḥammad ibn al-Ḥāriṯ al-Ḫušanī (mort en 361/971–972) a terminé à la demande d'al-Ḥakam II une histoire de juges de Cordoue. Muḥammad ibn al-Ḥasan al-Zubaydī (mort en 379/989–990) a écrit des *Ṭabaqāt* de grammairiens dont le dernier chapitre est consacré aux Andalous. Il s'agit de montrer que par leur nombre et leur qualité les savants andalous sont capables de rivaliser avec ceux de l'Orient", see GueṬab 51; and Miquel Forcada makes a similar point, saying: "Es bien sabido que la obra biográfica de Ibn Ŷulŷul aparece en un momento especialmente propicio para el género. Dada la profusión de obras análogas, podría parecer que se trata del capítulo médico de una enciclopedia biográfica andalusí compuesta además por el *Taʾrīj quḍāt Qurṭuba* de al-Jušanī (m. 371/981), las *Ṭabaqāt al-naḥwiyyīn wa-l-lugawiyyīn* de al-Zubaydī (m. 379/989) y el *Taʾrīj ʿulamāʾ al-Andalus* de Ibn al-Faraḍī (m. 403/1013), por citar sólo las que han llegado a nosotros", see ForBC 203 f.

66 Cf. Manfred Ullmann's remark that "[Ibn Ǧulǧul] wendete die literarische Darstellungsform der Klassifizierung nach Generationen, die in den Biographien der Traditionarier

related to the problem of genre prototypes is that of *topical* precursors. We already had occasion, in the course of examining Ibn Juljul's sources, to give a few hints in that direction,[67] and we shall address in the following subsection the question of how he handled them. Suffice it here to repeat that the only topical precursor to which Ibn Juljul might conceivably have had direct access is Isḥāq ibn Ḥunayn's (d. 298/910) so-called *Taʾrīkh al-aṭibbāʾ* "History of Physicians", a work that itself appears to be based largely on a now lost Greek writing by the Byzantine scholar Ioannes Philoponos (d. ca. 570 CE), also known as John the Grammarian (Arabic: Yaḥyā l-Naḥwī).[68] A copy of Isḥāq ibn Ḥunayn's small work[69] may well have reached Ibn Juljul together with the other medical and scientific books from the East which he himself says arrived in al-Andalus during the reign of ʿAbd al-Raḥmān III, that is around the middle of the 4th/10th century.[70] However, and not even dwelling on the extreme brevity of Isḥāq's *History*, it is important to remember that, first, this writing is mainly concerned with the primordial origins of medicine and an Old Testament-style chronology of principal physicians, running from Asclepius through Galen to Ioannes Philoponos, and ending with a coarse chronological concordance involving Adam, Moses and Jesus; second, and in the present context perhaps most crucially, Isḥāq's *History*, though organized chronologically, makes almost no attempt at providing *biographical* information proper, and therefore qualifies as an exponent of the *ṭabaqāt* genre only in the very broadest of terms.

3.3.3 Handling of Sources

Apart from a few pieces of information which Ibn Juljul obtained through *oral* transmissions and which he tends to indicate as such,[71] his source mater-

---

ihren Ursprung hatte und dann auch die Biographien der Dichter beherrschte, zum erstenmal auf die Medizingeschichte an", see UllMed 230.

67 Cf. p. 8 above with note 42.

68 See RoTA 56 f. with GaS 3/159 no. 1; further VerMA 450. On Ioannes/Yaḥyā cf. WilJP and WisYN *passim*.

69 For an Arabic edition and English translation (totalling 20 pages!) see RoTA 61–80.

70 See p. 93 below (end of biography 40).

71 Cf. pp. 9 f. above with note 55. Consider here in passing Juan Vernet's perhaps not altogether idle observations that Ibn Juljul could have obtained valuable pieces of information about Greek scholars directly from the Byzantine monk Nikolaos (cf. note 18 above) and others in his circle (?); that at least colloquial Greek was likely spoken/understood by a number of local merchants, travellers and government secretaries (?); and that some Mozarab clerics might have produced Romance language versions of Ibn Juljul's Latin sources, which then would have been linguistically accessible to him (?), see VerMA 452.

ial can be divided linguistically into three original strands: Greek, Latin, and Arabic.[72] As it is certain that Ibn Juljul knew no Greek,[73] and almost certain that he knew no Latin either,[74] he must have used these two strands of written sources in the form of Arabic translations. Here, all *Greek* texts which he explicitly or implicitly cites had been translated into Arabic in the Islamic East during the second half of the 3rd/9th century, and they very likely had made their way to al-Andalus by the middle of the 4th/10th century, if not earlier;[75] Arabic translations of *Latin* texts, insofar as they are referred to by Ibn Juljul, were no doubt produced exclusively in Muslim Spain, and probably during the first half of the 4th/10th century;[76] his genuinely *Arabic* sources, as far as they are identifiable, are of eastern provenance. Before we concentrate on the main question, it may be worth mentioning en passant that Ibn Juljul, just like his eastern peers, shows no particular interest in what was called 'prophetic medicine', even though a local literary specimen of that branch—al-Malik ibn Ḥabīb al-Qurṭubī's (d. 238/852) *Mukhtaṣar fī l-ṭibb*[77]—must have been right before his eyes,[78] and even though in his youth he, too, was a student of Muslim traditions (*ḥadīth*). It has already been indicated that Ibn Juljul, for the biographies of his Andalusian fellows (35–57), appears to have relied largely on common knowledge and direct informants; any *texts* that, in theory, he may additionally have had at his disposal are

---

72 See p. 9 above.

73 He himself states, in the introduction to his *Explanation of the Names of Simple Drugs in the Book of Dioscorides* (p. 5 above no. 2), that in the middle of the 4th/10th century, before the arrival of Nikolaos (cf. note 18 above), nobody in Córdoba, not even among the Christians, was able to read *ancient* Greek (*lam yakun yawma'idh*[in] *bi-Qurṭuba min naṣārā l-Andalus man yaqra'u l-lisān al-ighrīqī lladhī huwa l-yūnānī l-qadīm* [IAU 2.2/929,5 f.])—a verdict which, one must assume, included himself.

74 There is no indication—not in the *Generations* nor in any other of Ibn Juljul's extant works—that he was so much as rudimentarily familiar with the Latin language.

75 Cf. p. 93 below (end of biography 40). In the footnotes to our present translation, we are throughout specifying both the Greek work titles and the Arabic adaptations of that cluster of texts.

76 For a concise general survey of this track of transmission see VerOO 84–88. Note here also Ibn Juljul's own, broad-brush observation that up until the middle of the 3rd/9th century, medicine in al-Andalus was practised (only?) by Christians, who relied in this regard on a book which he calls *(al-)Aburīshim*, a transliterated term that suggests a Latin (or Old Castilian) intermediate form of Ἀφορισμοί, see pp. 88 f. below (preamble to chapter nine).

77 Cf. GaS 3/230 and ForBC 216.

78 The fact that on two occasions Ibn Juljul clearly did fish in the 'medical' chapters of one or another traditionist writing (cf. biographies 16 and 17) is, in my opinion, primarily due to his penchant for anecdotes, which, for the earliest period of Islamic history, he would only have found in this type of literature.

no longer tangible. For his biographies of non-Andalusians (1–34) he obviously relied on written sources, which latter Miquel Forcada has characterized as "poorly suited" to the task[79]—statements like this, however, confuse to some extent the issue of suitability with the problem of availability, as though Ibn Juljul, at the time and in the place he was writing, would have had much of a choice. Any attempt, then, at assessing Ibn Juljul's handling of written sources must take into account the fact that whichever writing he was able to use might have presented itself to him in a textual shape different from the one we possess today—this is particularly true for his quotations from Arabic translations of Greek and Latin works which he may well have seen in compositional casts involving abridgements, amplifications, reformulations, stealth commentaries, and even titular or authorial misattributions. Looking at Ibn Juljul's quotations from *Greek* sources, a corresponding picture emerges.[80]

The following short table illustrates both the paucity and the presumable defectiveness of the Greek sources which Ibn Juljul was able (or inclined) to cite. We do, of course, have no idea about how much stuff of that kind might have been around in Muslim Spain at the time; but if the below findings are anything to go by, and if we extrapolate them onto a larger canvas, the gap between what seems to have been available to Ibn Juljul, on the one hand, and the sheer volume of Greek medico-philosophical texts which were available in translations to his contemporaries in the Islamic East, on the other hand, cannot be imagined to be more dramatic.[81]

79 ForBC 211: "Desde el punto de vista de la información que contienen, estas biografías revelan la poca idoneidad de las fuentes que el autor maneja para la confección de un repertorio biográfico completo, ya sea por demasiado generales [...] o, al contrario, por demasiado específicas y ajenas al género histórico o biográfico [...] Con estos mimbres algo escasos confecciona unas biografías que, comparadas con otras fuentes, resultan desiguales e incompletas".

80 Not included here are the pseudo-Platonic *Laws* and the pseudo-Aristotelian *Secret of Secrets*, both of which are genuinely Arabic productions dating to the 3rd/9th and 4th/10th centuries (mistaken for the originals in ŶulGen 19, A-6 and A-8). It also goes without saying that the number of Greek works which Ibn Juljul knew *by title* through Ḥunayn ibn Isḥāq's Galen-bibliography would have been much larger, cf. p. 8 above with note 44.

81 A mere glance at the relevant bio-bibliographical chapters in Ibn al-Nadīm's *al-Fihrist* "The Catalogue" will readily confirm this observation, see NadFih 1/238–303; Ibn al-Nadīm was a Baghdad bookdealer who completed his *Catalogue*, as chance would have it, in the very same year as Ibn Juljul completed his *Generations* (i.e. in 377/987), but it is almost certain that they knew nothing of each other, never mind of their respective literary projects.

Biography	Ibn Juljul's Quotation	Actual Source	Verifiable[82]	Unverifiable
4	Hippocrates *Ὅρκος*	ps-Hippocrates *Ποδαπὸν δεῖ εἶναι τὸν ἰατρόν*	○	
4	*idem*			○
4	*idem*			○
4	Galen *Προτρεπτικὸς ἐπ' ἰατρικήν*			○
4	Galen *Πρὸς Γλαύκωνα θεραπευτικά*	Galen *Θεραπευτικὴ μέθοδος*	○	
4	Galen *Θεραπευτικὴ μέθοδος*			○
4	Galen *s.t.*	ps-Galen *Εἰς τὸ Ἱπποκράτους περὶ ὅρκου*	○	
6	Hippocrates *Ὅρκος*	ps-Hippocrates *Ποδαπὸν δεῖ εἶναι τὸν ἰατρόν*	○	
6	Galen *Ὅτι ὁ ἄριστος ἰατρὸς καὶ φιλόσοφος*		○	
7	Galen *s.t.*	Galen *Περὶ κράσεως καὶ δυνάμεως τῶν ἁπλῶν φαρμάκων*	○	
15	Galen *Περὶ δυσιάτων νοσημάτων* (lost in Greek and Arabic)		–	–
15	Galen *Περὶ συνθέσεως φαρμάκων τῶν κατὰ γένη*		○	
15	Galen *Θεραπευτικὴ μέθοδος*			○
15	Galen *Miḥnat al-ṭabīb* (lost in Greek)		○	

As regards the *Latin* sources which Ibn Juljul sweepingly refers to and/or from which he scatteringly quotes, they are three: Saint Jerome's (d. 420 CE) *Chroni-*

82 Most 'verifiable' quotations are paraphrastic and/or heavily warped, which may be due to Ibn Juljul's *Vorlage*, or to himself, or to both. Note in this connection that on one occasion (end of biography **14**), Ibn Juljul explicitly highlights a *literal* quotation (… *ʿalā mā ḥakaytu naṣṣ[an]*).

cum (referred to in the prologue but not explicitly quoted from);[83] Paulus Orosius' (d. ca. 420 CE) *Historiae adversus paganos* (referred to in the prologue and subsequently quoted twice);[84] and Isidore of Seville's (d. 636 CE) *Origines* (i.q. *Etymologiae*, quoted once).[85] The first to emphasize the significance of these references was Fu'ād Sayyid, the editor of the Arabic text of Ibn Juljul's *Ṭabaqāt*, saying: "[Le livre] d'Ibn Ǧulǧul doit retenir l'attention, notamment parce qu'il utilise les traductions arabes d'ouvrages d'histoire composés en latin, ce qui lui confère un intérêt incomparable".[86] And Sayyid is right, as the incorporation of this strand of sources lends to Ibn Juljul's *Generations* the unique distinction of being the earliest (and one of only a few) Arabic writings that made use of Latin works at all; in fact, the very existence of such Latin-into-Arabic translations is, at least in two of the aforesaid three cases, known to us solely through Ibn Juljul's text. Thus, there is no other *clear-cut* reference to an Arabic translation of Saint Jerome's *Chronicle*[87] or Isidore of Seville's *Origins*,[88] whilst an Arabic translation of Paulus Orosius' *Histories* has fortunately come down to us.[89] With the exception of the latter writing, we therefore possess hardly any tools to assess the quality of these translations or, indeed, the way Ibn Juljul dealt with them; besides, what has been said above about the various possibilities of textual alienation in Greek sources applies no doubt also to the Latin sources. Since there are no direct quotations from Saint Jerome's *Chronicle*, Ibn Juljul's management of that source is impossible to gauge; as for Paulus Orosius' *Histories*, the first quotation (**4**) cannot be substantiated in either the extant Arabic nor, for that matter, Latin text of that work,[90] whilst the second, very short quotation (**12**) is traceable to the original;[91] lastly, the isolated quotation from Isidore of Seville's *Origins* (**15**) is not found in the Latin text of that work but may well reflect a secondary amplification (gloss) which might have been part of the now lost Arabic translation.[92]

---

83 Arabic form of reference: Yirūnim the translator (*al-tarjumān*), *al-Qurūniqa*, see p. 33 below with note 5; Jerome is mentioned again en passant in biography **12**.

84 Arabic form of reference: Hurūshyush, author (*ṣāḥib*) of *al-Qiṣaṣ*, see p. 32 below with note 4; for the quotations see biographies **4** and **12**.

85 Arabic form of reference: Ishīdur al-Ishbīlī the metropolitan (*al-muṭrān*), no work title given, see biography **15** with note 159.

86 JulṬab 5 (French introduction); cf. also ibid. pp. كط—له (Arabic introduction).

87 Latin text edition see bibliography s.n. HieCh.

88 Latin text edition see bibliography s.n. IsEty.

89 Latin text edition see bibliography s.n. OrHis; Arabic text editions s.nn. OrKit and OrTa'.

90 See p. 39 below with note 39.

91 See p. 54 below with note 135.

92 See p. 57 below with note 159.

As regards genuinely *Arabic* sources, Ibn Juljul explicitly quotes but four: Abū Yūsuf Yaʿqūb ibn Isḥāq al-Kindī's (d. ca. 256/870) *Risāla fī Aghrāḍ (kutub) Uqlīdis* "Epistle on the Objectives (of the books) of Euclid" (quoted in **14**); Abū Maʿshar Jaʿfar ibn Muḥammad al-Balkhī's (d. 272/886) *Kitāb al-Ulūf* "Book of the Thousands" (referred to in the prologue, then quoted twice in **1** and **2**); pseudo-Plato's *al-Nawāmīs* "The Laws", composed in the second half of the 3rd/9th century in the Islamic East and not to be mistaken for Plato's *Νόμοι* (quoted thrice in **4**); and pseudo-Aristotle's *Sirr al-asrār* "The Secret of Secrets", composed in the early 4th/10th century in the Islamic East (quoted in **9**).[93] With the exception of the latter work, these sources are now almost entirely lost, and one can only assume a more or less faithful representation of them on the part of Ibn Juljul; as for pseudo-Aristotle's *Secrets*, the passage quoted by Ibn Juljul is virtually identical with the extant Arabic text.[94] *Implicit* Arabic sources are suggested by fleeting references to the corpus of traditionist literature[95] as well as by one possible, though highly speculative implication of Sābūr ibn Sahl's (d. 255/869) pharmacopoeia (*aqrābādhīn*).[96]

Finally, I do not wish to conceal my bafflement about a Bible-quotation (*James* 1:17) which Ibn Juljul, a Muslim writing for a fellow Muslim, deemed worthy of incorporation into the prologue of his work.[97]

3.3.4 Selective Character

When looking at the list of biographed individuals in Ibn Juljul's *Generations*,[98] it is immediately obvious that whilst his choices far exceed in scope and ambition the largely computational register of Isḥāq ibn Ḥunayn,[99] they are at the same time considerably more restricted than, say, those made by his successors al-Qifṭī and Ibn Abī Uṣaybiʿa.[100] It is true that insofar as non-Andalusian scholars are concerned, this has a lot to do with the relatively scarce amount of sources which Ibn Juljul had at his disposal; and it is also true that Ibn Juljul himself, in the epilogue to his work, makes no secret of self-imposed restrictions and selective criteria. However, when running through his biographies

93 Another reference to this work in biography **23** reiterates the (legendary) involvement of Yūḥannā ibn al-Biṭrīq (fl. around 200/815) in its (legendary) 'translation'.

94 See BadUṣ 126 f.

95 Possibly (but by no means exclusively) Mālik ibn Anas' *al-Muwaṭṭaʾ* (**16**) and Aḥmad ibn Ḥanbal's *al-Musnad* (**17**).

96 See p. 94 below (biography **41** with note 430).

97 See p. 33 below with note 8.

98 See the table on pp. 10 ff. above.

99 Cf. RoTA 75–80.

100 For their works see bibliography s.nn. QifTa' and IAU, respectively.

of *Andalusian* scholars (35–57), and precisely by taking his declared limitations at face value,[101] a more problematic question arises, namely that of glaring omissions. The latter have been explained by some modern researchers as being politically motivated and/or the result of a professional bias on the part of Ibn Juljul—we will return to these points in the following subsection. Suffice it here to name a few striking examples of highly renowned, if not celebrated scholars who were Ibn Juljul's contemporaries and lived, like he did, in Córdoba, but whom he completely ignores: ʿArīb ibn Saʿīd, physician and polymath (d. ca. 370/980);[102] Abū Bakr Ḥāmid ibn Samajūn, physician and pharmacologist (d. ca. 390/1000);[103] Abū l-Qāsim al-Zahrāwī, physician and surgeon (d. soon after 399/1009);[104] and others still.[105] The same applies to the scholars who, according to Ibn Juljul's own account,[106] collaborated with him, for years, on the revision of the Arabic translation of Dioscorides' *Περὶ ὕλης ἰατρικῆς*: Nikolaos, the Byzantine monk;[107] Ḥasdāy Ibn Shaprūṭ, the Jewish court physician;[108] Muḥammad, known as al-Shajjār 'the botanist';[109] a certain al-Basbāsī;[110] Abū ʿUthmān al-Jazzār, nicknamed al-Yābisa 'terra firma' or, perhaps

101 He writes: "We concentrated on famous, well-known (and) accessible (men) from our homeland of al-Andalus, (who lived) under the guidance of leaders […] that pursued knowledge and strove for wisdom; we (further) narrowed our focus on naming those (among them) who served (the court), but not such of their contemporaries as were no match for them nor occupied an equally (important) position, worthy of being dealt with at any length" (*wa-ʾqtaṣarnā ʿalā man ʿarafnā bi-nāḥiyatinā bi-l-Andalus idh kānū mashhūrīna maʿrūfīna ẓāhirīna fī duwal aʾimmat*^{in} *lil-ʿilm ṭālibīna wa-ʿan al-ḥikma bāḥithīna* […] *wa-ʾqtaṣarnā ʿalā dhikr al-mashhūrīna l-ẓāhirīna l-khādimīna wa-aḍrabnā ʿan dhikr man kāna fī zamānihim mimman lam yuwāzihim wa-lā ḥalla maḥallahum idh lam yakūnū min ittisāʿ al-dhikr bi-maḥall hāʾulāʾ*), see pp. 109 f. below (epilogue) with JulṬab ١١٦,8–12.

102 On him see ForʿAS *passim*.

103 On him see VerIS *passim*.

104 On him see SSZah *passim*; note, however, that some more recent scholars postdate al-Zahrāwī's death by at least two decades, see JanNMD 1/168.

105 GueṬab 54 f. cites as further examples (after ṢAṬab 81 f.) the well-known physicians ʿAbdallāh ibn Isḥāq, aka Ibn al-Shanāʿa al-Muslimānī al-Isrāʾīlī (!); Abū ʿAbdallāh Muḥammad ibn al-Ḥusayn, aka Ibn al-Kattānī (the nephew of 50); and Abū l-ʿArab Yūsuf ibn Muḥammad.

106 *Apud* IAU 3.2/1039; cf. also UllMM 62.

107 Cf. note 18 above.

108 Cf. note 19 above.

109 Not further identifiable.

110 The translators of Ibn Abī Uṣaybiʿa's report suggest, against all manuscript evidence, to read al-Shabānisī (instead of al-Basbāsī), see IAU 3.2/1039 note 11; they refer to AbbTak 2/53 no. 1106, who gives a short biography of Muḥammad ibn Qāsim al-Qurashī *al-Sha/ibānisī* from Córdoba but does not say that the latter was "a physician"; more importantly, though, this al-Sha/ibānisī died in the year 447/1055, which renders any involvement on his part in the Dioscorides-revision (which began in the 340s/950s and lasted for about two decades)

more likely, ‘the withered (hand?)’;[111] Muḥammad ibn Saʿīd, the physician;[112] ʿAbd al-Raḥmān ibn Isḥāq ibn Haytham;[113] and Abū ʿAbdallāh, the Sicilian who spoke Greek.[114]

3.3.5 Compositional Intention

The overall textual makeup of Ibn Juljul’s *Generations* reflects a number of compositional peculiarities which go well beyond the *presumed* primary intention of transmitting information, whether factual or fictional. First, as we have just seen when looking at the idiosyncratic choices he made with regard to his *Andalusian* peers, there is a fair count of scholars whom he should have, but did not, honour with a biographical entry—these omissions cannot be explained by his declared ambition to be brief, nor by his almost cynical assertion that he prefers substance over prolixity.[115] Second, and unlike other medieval Arab biographers, Ibn Juljul makes no palpable effort and shows no particular concern to provide strictly chronological data, such as dates of birth and death, nor does he exhibit a sustained desire to place his subjects into a framework of teacher-pupil relations—instead, he is generally content to convey this kind of information by linking it to dynastic timelines, individual rulers or, in case of prehistoric/mythical ‘sages’ (**1–5**), to major events (the Flood) or to biblical figures.[116] Third, and perhaps most surprising in view of the aforesaid limitations, Ibn Juljul’s work is extraordinarily rich in anecdotal material, around which it almost seems to revolve—this trait illustrates more than anything else the fact that his intention was not focused above all on the transmission of factual information but rather on the composition of a literary specimen in the *adab* or

---

virtually impossible; besides, Ibn Juljul himself confirms (*apud* IAU 3.2/1039,-2) that this group of scholars all lived at the same time (*fī zamān wāḥid*).

111 The translators of Ibn Abī Uṣaybiʿa’s report suggest to emend the strange epithet al-Yābisa to read al-Yābisī ‘the Ibizan’, see IAU 3.2/1039 note 12. Also observe that UllMM 62,20 prefers the reading al-Ḥazzāz (over al-Jazzār), presumably by emending the lemma الجزاز which is attested as such in one of the manuscripts of Ibn Abī Uṣaybiʿa’s text, see IAU 2.2/930 note 20.

112 Not further identifiable.

113 Flourished second half of 4th/10th century, see GaS 3/314.

114 Not further identifiable.

115 Thus, he writes: “We chose quality over quantity so as not to exhaust the reader’s patience, and to make it easier for the mind to retain (the information)—for overmuch talking is hard to bear” (*wa-ʾqtaṣarnā ʿalā qalīl min kathīr li-allā yamallahū qāriʾuhū wa-li-yashula ʿalā l-nafs ḥifẓuhū wa-l-kalām idhā ṭāla thaqula*), see p. 110 below (epilogue) with JulṬab ١١٦,13f.

116 In this connection, Miquel Forcada reminds us that Ibn Juljul was neither a trained historian nor a practised biographer, cf. ForBC 208.

belletristic vein,[117] including burlesque mockery and borderline gossip. Fourth, it is also important to consider here Ibn Juljul's pronouncement that he wrote the work at the request of an (unnamed) nobleman,[118] as well as his idea to append to it a (now lost) autobiographical survey.[119]

All these features, overlapping and intertwining, make it very difficult to formulate a unified theory about the compositional intention behind Ibn Juljul's *Generations*, and it is no wonder that the few scholars who have so far engaged at all with the problem of the work's purpose and aim, drew different, sometimes incompatible conclusions. Perhaps the most original, albeit quite reductive interpretation on record is that proposed in 1992 by Marie-Geneviève Guesdon. In a nutshell, it goes like this: Ibn Juljul's work, completed in 377/987, is an indirect condemnation of the regime of the grand vizier Ibn Abī ʿĀmir al-Maʿāfirī (aka Almanzor), who had become the *de facto* ruler of al-Andalus a decade earlier, in 368/978, at the expense of the child-caliph Hishām II (reg. nominally from 366/976); under the preceding caliphs, ʿAbd al-Raḥmān III (reg. 316/929–350/961) and al-Ḥakam II (reg. 350/961–366/976), Córdoba had been a beacon of learning, whereas Almanzor was hostile to scientific and philosophical activities, ordered books to be burned, and tolerated only the pursuit of medicine and mathematics; the Andalusian scholars whom Ibn Juljul 'omitted' to incorporate into his work were all associated with, if not directly serving, Almanzor; the unnamed addressee in Ibn Juljul's prologue is a member of the (disenfranchised) Umayyad house; Ibn Juljul's statement that the usurpation of power in the Islamic East by "the Daylamites and the Turks" led to cultural decline, and his explicit focus on those Andalusian scholars who lived "under the guidance of leaders [...] that pursued knowledge and strove for wisdom",[120] are to be seen as a disguised but direct invitation to contemplate the course of Almanzor's career and his intellectual attitudes; Ibn Juljul's work therefore offers a critique of the transition of power from a legitimate and nourishing to an illegitimate and repressive form of government; as such, it is an essentially political piece of writing.[121]

A few years later, in 1997, Miquel Forcada, without disputing the above line of interpretation, puts no less a stronger emphasis on the facts that Ibn Juljul's work is, first, the immediate product of a commission (by an "Umayyad prince") and, second, largely anecdotal in its literary character, which suggests a core

117 This is why the work has once been described as "casi un anecdotario", see ForBC 206,19.
118 See p. 31 below (beginning of prologue).
119 See p. 110 below (end of epilogue).
120 See p. 109 below (epilogue).
121 Cf. GueṬab *passim*.

function of entertainment;[122] however, Forcada remains highly sceptical about the possibilities of disentangling Ibn Juljul's intentions.[123]

Lastly, Cristina Álvarez Millán, in a superb article from 2004, begins by driving home a few commonsensical observations, namely that medico-biographical dictionaries, regardless of any claims they may make about providing historical facts, also always have a social function and constitute, through their more or less ample incorporation of anecdotal material, invariably a part of *adab* or belletristic literature; further, the role of book-writing as a means of self-promotion, especially among the medical profession, needs to be taken into account.[124] The most interesting aspect of her study, insofar as our current purposes are concerned, is Álvarez Millán's strong opposition to Guesdon's claim that Ibn Juljul's work represents a condemnation of ʿĀmirid power: by analyzing in detail the drift of Ibn Juljul's biographical entries of *Andalusian* scholars (35–57), she shows that the number of 'negative' (i.e. critical or pejorative) biographies[125] is higher under the reigns he is allegedly defending; by the same token, Ibn Juljul's omission of the group of scholars who collaborated, during the reign of ʿAbd al-Raḥmān III, on the revision of the Dioscorides-codex,[126] can be viewed as an act of literary sabotage against physicians that were associated with this ruler. In short, according to Álvarez Millán, the inner features of Ibn Juljul's work suggest that its recipient (scil. addressee) was Almanzor himself instead, whose favour Ibn Juljul might thereby have tried to gain or to retain.[127]

Whilst I cannot, unfortunately, contribute any new ideas to this discussion, I should nonetheless like to point out that it is *generally* rather difficult to narrow down, never mind clearly identify, authorial intentions in medieval Arabic lit-

122 Cf. ForBC 204–209.

123 "Ante la imposibilidad de realizar un juicio sobre las intenciones de Ibn Ŷulŷul, resulta difícil contrastar la bondad de las opiniones expuestas", see ForBC 206,12 ff.; similarly ÁlMiIŶ 68b,24 f.: "No está clara, por tanto, la intención del autor al escribir esta obra".

124 Cf. ÁlMiBD 142 ff. Here, the fact that Ibn Juljul, rather unusually, appended his own 'CV' to the *Ṭabaqāt* is considered by Álvarez Millán as an attempt to highlight his professional credentials and enhance his medical authority, cf. ibid. 155.

125 Including snobbery and self-indulgence (35), greed (37), secretiveness (44), stinginess (46), homosexuality/pederasty (45 and 47), and gluttony (53).

126 Cf. pp. 21 f. above.

127 Cf. ÁlMiBD 152 ff. Note in passing that Álvarez Millán also opposes Guesdon's concomitant claim about Ibn Juljul's book, namely that it may represent a (chauvinistic) refutation of the perceived but bygone superiority of *eastern* Islamic scholars—this interpretation, too, makes no sense in Álvarez Millán's view, who points to the "deplorable panorama" which Ibn Juljul paints with regard to his chosen *Andalusian* protagonists, see ÁlMiBD 153,ult.–154,3.

erary productions, not least because there is often no harmonious correlation between subject matter and presentational style; and the more a given piece of writing tilts towards the *adab* genre, the murkier the problem becomes. As regards the elusive question of the *addressee*, I am inclined to think that we are looking here, most likely, at a person closely related to the caliph Hishām II—for would Ibn Juljul have described Almanzor, who despite his old and purely Arab lineage was basically a parvenu, as someone "of good Umayyad and Qurayshite stock, scion of caliphs, descendant of imams heralding the true religion"?[128]

3.3.6 Residual Impact

If Ibn Juljul's pronouncement that he composed his *Generations* at the request of an Arab nobleman[129] is a reflection of real events, then it may well be that the work initially had a very limited circulation.[130] In the years, decades and centuries that followed, however, Ibn Juljul's book must have gained a certain popularity, first among like-minded writers (that is to say biographers) in al-Andalus, but subsequently also among intellectuals of the Islamic East.[131] Thus, the Toledan judge Ṣāʿid ibn Aḥmad al-Andalusī (d. 462/1070) amply used Ibn Juljul's book in his own *Ṭabaqāt al-umam* "Layers of Nations",[132] and through the latter some of its content also entered the biographical works of the Andalusians al-Ḥumaydī (d. 488/1095), Ibn Bashkuwāl (d. 578/1183), al-Ḍabbī (d. 599/1203), and Ibn al-Abbār (d. 658/1260).[133] In the Islamic East, with considerable delay, Ibn Juljul's book became known to the biographer al-Qifṭī (d. 646/1248) who, judging from his own short characterization of it, must have actually possessed a copy,[134] whilst al-Dhahabī (d. 749/1348) had

---

128 See p. 33 below (end of prologue). Eloísa Llavero Ruiz, too, considers the addressee to be "uno de los nobles omeyas que vivieron en al-Andalus durante [la] época", see ŶulGen 109 note 1.

129 See p. 31 below (beginning of prologue).

130 That said, it is of course true that Ibn Juljul, between the completion of the *Generations* in 377/987 and his death after 384/994, would have been well placed, as a physician of the caliph, to advertise his book to the many scholars who regularly went in and out of the court.

131 Note, though, that only a single (North African) Arabic manuscript of Ibn Juljul's *Ṭabaqāt* has come down to us, cf. note 35 above.

132 See bibliography s.n. ṢAṬab and, for a short general assessment, ForBC 217,13–16 with note 48. It is likely that already Ibn al-Faraḍī (d. 403/1013) consulted, for the composition of his own *Taʾrīkh ʿulamāʾ al-Andalus* "History of the Scholars of al-Andalus", Ibn Juljul's *Generations*, cf. bibliography s.n. FarTaʾ.

133 See bibliography s.nn. AbbTak, BashṢi, ḌabbBu and ḤumJM; cf. also ForBC 238–241.

134 QifTaʾ 190,5 ff. (cf. note 25 above).

at least heard of it;[135] yet it was Ibn Abī Uṣaybiʿa (d. 668/1270) who, in his medico-biographical chef-d'œuvre, extracted from Ibn Juljul's book numerous passages, often verbatim, commencing with Apollo(n) (5) and going all the way to Muḥammad ibn ʿAbdūn al-Jabalī (57).[136] Considering the modest size and somewhat idiosyncratic literary character of Ibn Juljul's book, the fact that a towering figure like Ibn Abī Uṣaybiʿa, a Syrian who wrote almost 300 years later in a different part of the world, valued it enough to make hay with it, is by itself a remarkable token of both impact and appreciation. A systematic and detailed investigation into the transmissional fate of Ibn Juljul's *Generations*—well beyond the scope of our present work—must remain a task for the future.

3.3.7 Historical Substance

The historicity of the information transmitted by Ibn Juljul in his *Generations* should, first of all, not be confused with the work's historical significance. Second, any evaluation of its factual content has to take into account some largely open questions regarding compositional intention, which latter does not seem to have consisted primarily in the transmission of facts; directly linked to this problem is the author's penchant for communicating bribes of information in the form of anecdotal embedments[137]—in other words, we are looking here at both an imponderably biased chronicle and a cheerfully decorated exponent of entertainment literature. Next, and obviously, we need to exclude from historical scrutiny those biographed individuals that we, unlike Ibn Juljul, can safely consign to the realm of myth.[138] Finally, we have to distinguish between information that Ibn Juljul would have found relatively difficult to obtain from a limited number of more or less relevant texts (the 'Ancients' and the 'Easterners'), and information that he could have gathered from written sources closer to home, if not orally from contemporaneous witnesses (the 'Maghrebinians' and the 'Andalusians'). Having said that, there is a fair number of chronological, geographical and conceptual blunders in Ibn Juljul's *Generations*, even by the relatively modest standards of comparable medieval Arabic works of this literary genre. A few examples: a) *chronological* errors: Hippocrates and Polemon are considered contemporaries (6), Saint Jerome and Ptolemy II (or Claudius Ptolemy) are considered contemporaries (12), Galen

135 DhaTI 8/676,12 (cf. note 25 above).

136 IAU 2.1/56 = 3.1/53 (explicit) through to 2.2/926 f. = 3.2/1035 (implicit), and *passim* in between.

137 Cf. the discussion on pp. 22 ff. above.

138 That is, biographies 1–5 (Hermes I–III, Asclepius, and Apollon).

and Nero (or Tiberius) are considered contemporaries (**15**), Bukhtīshūʿ ibn Jurjīs is associated with the caliphs Abū l-ʿAbbās al-Saffāḥ and Abū Jaʿfar al-Manṣūr bi-llāh (**20** and **21**), the military campaigns against Ancyra and Amorium are associated with Hārūn al-Rashīd (**22**), Ḥunayn ibn Isḥāq is considered a pupil of al-Khalīl ibn Aḥmad (**24**); b) *geographical* errors: Cos is considered a city and equated with Homs (**6**), Pergamon is considered an island (as well as a city) (**15**), al-Khalīl ibn Aḥmad is said to have lived in Persia (**24**); c) *conceptual* errors: Dioscorides is said to have interpreted (lit. "translated") the writings of Hippocrates (**7**), Asclepius *and* Aristotle were "lifted up in a shaft of light" and *both* were called "angels rather than men" by God (**4** and **9**), Socrates is once confused (implicitly) with Diogenes (**10**), Ptolemy the pharaoh is confused with Ptolemy the scientist (**12**), Euclid is said to have explained the work of Apollonius (instead of vice versa) (**14**). Mistakes such as these are, no doubt, a direct result of the poor quality (and quantity) of the written sources which Ibn Juljul could access;[139] yet whilst we may reasonably suspect a somehow biased representation with regard to the *Andalusian* biographies, there is no reason whatsoever to assume that this is also true for the rest.[140] A different matter altogether is the thorny question of whether we will, at some point, be able to identify more clearly and follow more closely the still blurry tracks of transmission of late antique knowledge from the Islamic East to Muslim Spain.[141]

3.3.8 Epistemological Value

It is clear from the preceding disquisitions that Ibn Juljul's book represents very much a production *sui generis*. Whilst its formal structure and literary genre are relatively easy to describe and define, the manner in which the author handled

139 Cf. p. 9 above.

140 Other items of information, whose potential veracity has yet to be explored, include, for example: the Alexandrian physician Anqīlāwus is said to have orchestrated the redaction of the *Summaria Alexandrinorum*, and to have contributed himself thirteen of its sixteen parts (**ch.5** [intra]) (accepted as a fact GaS 3/160); the Syro-Persian Jew Māsarjawayh is said to have translated the medical compendium of Ahrun from Syriac into Arabic (**19**) (considered doubtful UllMed 23); and al-Kindī, called "a Basran" (?), is said to have written a couple of otherwise unattested works (**25**).

141 This prospect was already raised, perhaps overoptimistically, more than half a century ago by Manfred Ullmann, who wrote: "Die Nachrichten Ibn Ǧulǧuls über die antiken Ärzte weichen oft von der historischen Wahrheit ab; aber gerade die Fehler sind die Leitfäden, an Hand derer die Traditionswege des spätantiken Wissens aufgedeckt und nachgezeichnet werden können", see UllMed 230. Based on the textual tools we possess today, this task still remains largely elusive.

his unusual and scanty sources, the principles which guided his selection of material, as well as the oblique intentions which contributed to the works final form are much more difficult to pin down. A fairly sharp distinction can be made between the biographies of 'ancient' and non-Andalusian individuals (1–34), on the one hand, and those of Andalusians (35–57), on the other hand: the latter biographies are based, regardless of possible authorial proclivities and insinuations, on *local* knowledge, whether written down, commonly circulating or, as in several cases, obtained directly from oral informants. This also means that any data which we, in turn, may obtain from the 'Andalusian' part of Ibn Juljul's book are likely to be more reliable and to carry a higher degree of validity,[142] at least theoretically. The information he spreads out before us in regard to Greek and eastern Islamic "physicians and sages", insofar as they are not mythical altogether, is characterized by a striking eclecticism that at times verges into dilettantism; yet still it is very hard to tell whether this feature is due to the poverty and potential corruption of Ibn Juljul's sources, or to his own desire to narrow down and bend items of information into 'entertaining' shapes, or both. Consequently, there are hardly any new insights for us when it comes to the Greeks or, indeed, the eastern Islamic protagonists—all of which solidifies the impression that Ibn Juljul's book, independent of his own perhaps broader knowledge base, was conceived first and foremost as a historico-belletristic repository of vaguely educational (and sometimes moralizing) tales.

3.4 *Conclusion*

Looking back from a distance at the manifold facets of Ibn Juljul's *Generations of Physicians and Sages*, it is easy to see both the originality and the unwieldiness of this work within its given temporal, geographical, cultural and linguistic setting. His book is one of the earliest of its kind in Arabic literature. It offers a history of healers and seekers, of scientists and philosophers, legendary and real, from the dawn of days down to the author's immediate present, but it is, for all that, remarkably short and highly selective. The biographed *non-Andalusians*—Greeks and Arabs, Muslims, Christians and Jews, 'Easterners', Egyptians and Maghrebinians, from "before the Flood" to the time of Ibn Juljul—count only thirty-four in number and are allocated only about

142 Miquel Forcada summarized it nicely by saying: "Como ya he avanzado, a pesar de todas las limitaciones que el autor se impone, el libro de Ibn Ŷulŷul es el pilar fundamental de la historia de la medicina andalusí para el periodo que abarca, y la prueba de ello es el escaso número de médicos que quedan fuera de las *Ṭabaqāt*", see ForBC 215,8–12.

60% of the overall space; the *Andalusians*—Muslims and Christians, from the middle of the 3rd/9th to the second half of the 4th/10th centuries—count twenty-three in number and are allocated about 40%. Many of the historical 'facts' which the work aspires to transmit are bound up and presented as anecdotal parcels contrived to charm as much as to enlighten the reader, who at the time of its conception would have been a high-ranking Arab Muslim courtier or else a powerful politician. Ibn Juljul expresses himself in clear, albeit somewhat quaint and mannered classical Arabic, which testifies to an early exposure or, indeed, native competence in that language. Yet his general style of writing is characterized by repetition; the flow of his narrative is sometimes smooth and sometimes rough, unsteady, as though he had been intermittently drafting or repeatedly shelving and unshelving his drafts; and the impression on the whole is that of a not quite finished, rather erratic, almost inchoate piece of perhaps overly ambitious design. Ibn Juljul's choice to cast his material into the traditional *ṭabaqāt* format must have naturally presented itself to him and was certainly not hindered by the fact that he himself had been a student of *ḥadīth* literature, the quintessential vessel of this scholarly genre. Faced with the difficult and ultimately unanswerable question of what exactly Ibn Juljul may have *intended to achieve* by putting together a biographical inventory of that eclectic kind and conceptual drift, we cannot but view it from our own place in time, whence it appears to be a truly hybrid historical document: it paints a vivid and presumably authentic picture of Andalusian medicine in the 3rd/9th and notably 4th/10th centuries, whilst displaying an almost mystified attitude towards the Ancients; it employs rare, one-off Arabic translations of Latin sources, whilst suffering from a dire lack of Greco-Arabic texts which, in the Islamic East, were plentiful; and it insists on transmitting information largely in the guise of tales, which lends to the work a character of both fragmentation and tangibility.[143] In the end, it is to be hoped that the present, annotated English translation of Ibn Juljul's book does justice to the original and conveys to the modern reader not only historical insights but also at least some of its literary flavour.

---

143 Cf. also Eloísa Llavero Ruiz's concluding remark to her Spanish translation of Ibn Juljul's *Ṭabaqāt*: "En cuanto a la obra de Ibn Ŷulŷul, hay que hacer hincapié, una vez más, en que no es un tratado de medicina, ni tampoco una historia de los médicos en el sentido estricto, ya que algunos de los biografiados ocupan solamente un par de renglones sin apenas contenido biográfico. El interés de la misma radica, principalmente, en la recopilación de no pocas anécdotas, que, a veces, no aparecen en otras fuentes", see ŶulGen 107.

4 Plate

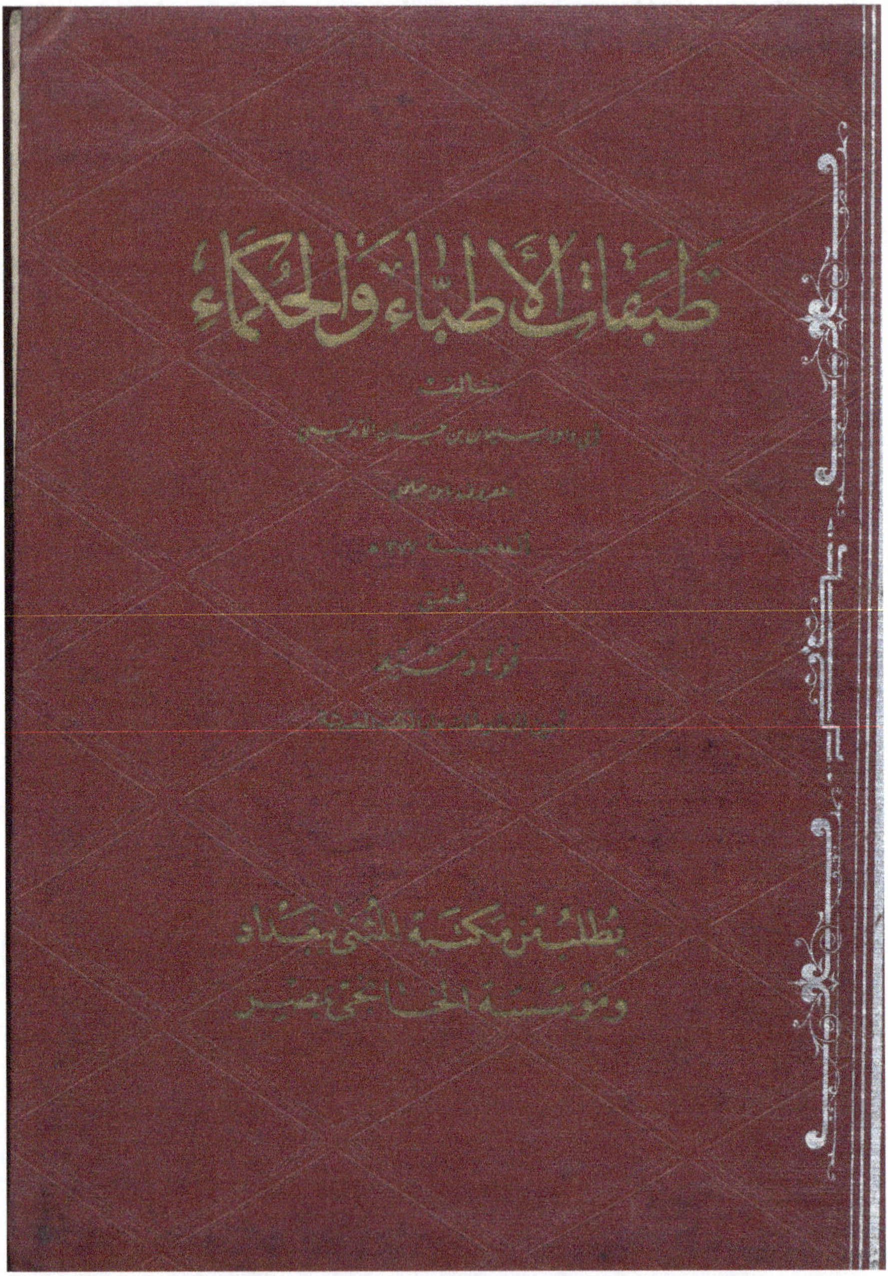

Cover of the Arabic edition of Ibn Juljul's *Generations of Physicians and Sages*, Cairo 1955

Translation

﴿١﴾ In the name of God the Merciful the Compassionate—
may He bless our lord Muḥammad, his family and his companions,
and grant [them] salvation!

Sulaymān ibn Ḥassān the healer—may God have mercy upon him—says:

You[*] asked, O learned Sire,[1] that I record for you the information I acquired by studying the books of past writers and the biographies of those who have gone before us, from the first who conceived of the art of medicine and spoke about it in the beginning of time, prior to the Flood and thereafter; further, in which

---

* The task of furnishing my translation with sufficiently detailed explanatory notes was greatly facilitated by being able to draw on the excellent commentary which Fu'ād Sayyid, the editor of Ibn Juljul's *Ṭabaqāt*, appended to each section of the Arabic text—readers familiar with this language are encouraged to continue using Sayyid's erudite annotations, especially with regard to the wealth of auxiliary source documentation which would largely be lost on non-Arabic speakers. In order to ease the navigation between Arabic and English text, I have inserted ornate parentheses into my translation, showing the pagination of Sayyid's edition; moreover, each biographical entry is structured so as to match both the section numbering and overall textual layout of the Arabic. Many passages from Ibn Juljul's *Ṭabaqāt* were quoted, more or less literally, by Ibn Abī Uṣaybiʿa (d. 668/1270) in his medical history titled *ʿUyūn al-anbāʾ*—here, it has always been instructive to be able to juxtapose such passages with the new Arabic edition and annotated English translation of Ibn Abī Uṣaybiʿa's work (see bibliography s.n. IAU). Eloísa Llavero Ruiz's complete Spanish translation of Ibn Juljul's *Ṭabaqāt* from 1979 (see bibliography s.n. ŶulGen), including a concise introduction and multiple notes, has been considered throughout; any additional (and still relevant) prefatory and explanatory remarks she made have been worked into the introduction and into all footnotes of the present book; note that Llavero Ruiz did not trouble herself with source verifications, nor with the compilation of an index. For the last chapter of the *Ṭabaqāt* (biographies 35–57), Juan Vernet's Spanish translation from 1968 (see bibliography s.n. VerMA), though somewhat hastily executed, offered no less a few interesting points of comparison. Finally, by way of a general remark, it may be worth noting that Ibn Juljul, especially in the early sections of his book, uses three different terms to signify "Greek": *yūnānī*, *rūmī* and *ghirīqī*—strictly speaking, in medieval Arabic, *(al-)Yūnān* (< *Ἴωνες* "Ionians") denotes the Ancient Greeks, *(al-)Rūm* (< *Ῥωμαῖοι* "Romæans") denotes the 'Eastern Romans' or Byzantine Greeks but sometimes also the Romans, and *(al-)Ghirīqiyyūn* (< Latin *Græci* < *Γραικοί*) denotes the 'Western (i.e. homeland) Greeks'; however, Ibn Juljul does not seem to employ these terms in a consistent, logical or even intentional fashion, and I have therefore allowed myself a certain leeway in their translation, proceeding on a case-by-case basis.

1 The unnamed nobleman whom Ibn Juljul addresses here and elsewhere in his prologue, and upon whose instigation he professes to have composed the present book, could have

© KONINKLIJKE BRILL NV, LEIDEN, 2023 | DOI:10.1163/9789004682238_003

era each protagonist lived whose name is well known[2] and whose reputation widespread, whose skill has proven itself, whose wisdom has endured, and who made a lasting contribution, worthy of recognition.

You mentioned that you have not seen a satisfactory book nor a persuasive, detailed account on any of those predecessors, which is why I felt obliged to respond to your request and to meet your desire—for in this [matter], I do indeed possess what I hope should disperse your doubt and sufficiently enlighten you, God willing. With this epistle of mine, I also intend to revive the story of some of those whose memory has faded and whose vestige been effaced, but I am only communicating to you, O Sire, such [items of] information that I myself obtained through examining and exploring ﴾٢﴿ the ancient writings, like the *Book of the Thousands* of Abū Maʿshar the astrologer,[3] or like the book of Orosius ﴾٣﴿ the author of *The Histories*,[4] or like the book [titled]

been a relative or courtier of the caliph Abū l-Walīd Hishām II ibn al-Ḥakam al-Mu'ayyad bi-llāh (reg. 366/976–399/1009 and, after a brief interlude, again from 400/1010–403/1013), whom Ibn Juljul served as personal physician; possible also is that the person in question was Muḥammad ibn ʿAbdallāh Ibn Abī ʿĀmir al-Maʿāfirī, known as al-Manṣūr bi-llāh (*Almanzor* in Spanish chronicles), a landowning Arab aristocrat who rose to be chancellor, chamberlain and *de facto* ruler of al-Andalus from 368/978 until his death in 392/1002, see on him CPPL 14–53 with ChMan *passim*. At the end of his prologue, Ibn Juljul describes the high-ranking personage as a man "of good Umayyad and Qurayshite stock, scion of caliphs, descendant of imams heralding the true religion". Cristina Álvarez Millán rightly points out that Ibn Juljul's claim, namely that he composed his book in response to a request, may be interpreted simply as a literary topos (ÁlMiBD 147 f.); yet she, too, raises the possibility that the addressee of the work might be the aforesaid al-Manṣūr bi-llāh (ibid. 154). On the other hand, Marie-Geneviève Guesdon, following her own interpretive logic, considers the addressee to be a member of the Umayyad house (GueṬab 59; likewise ForBC 204,14: "un príncipe omeya"). Any attempt at answering this challenging question is intrinsically linked to the postulation of a distinct politico-cultural agenda on the part of Ibn Juljul—cf. pp. 22–25 above for a discussion of the problem.

2 Read *shīʿa* (instead of *shuniʿa*).

3 Abū Maʿshar Jaʿfar ibn Muḥammad al-Balkhī (d. 272/886), a famous Arabic-writing astrologer of Persian descent, on whose life, works and influence see e.g. PinAM *passim* and, most recently, YaBuAM 1/1–6; his *Kitāb al-Ulūf* or "Book of the Thousands", a work on astrological history, is preserved today only in the form of a short summary whose content, and especially mathematical material, has been studied monographically by David Pingree, see PinTAM 13–27, 57–68 and *passim*.

4 Paulus Orosius (Arabic *Hurūshyush*, d. ca. 420 CE), a Roman priest and historian from Braga in modern-day Portugal, is the author of a famous, much-read universal history titled *Historiae adversus paganos*, which was subsequently translated into several languages; an Arabic translation, based on a 7th-century CE Latin redaction and referred to here by Ibn Juljul as *al-Qiṣaṣ* or "The Histories", was made in Córdoba by a small group of Christian scholars (involving Ḥafṣ ibn Albar 'the Goth' and Qāsim ibn Aṣbagh 'the judge') during the second quarter of the 4th/10th century on behalf of the prince and future caliph al-Ḥakam II (b. 302/915, reg.

The Chronicle of Jerome the translator,[5] or like the reports I have seen concerning sages of the Greek realm[6]—from these [sources] I was able to infer each man's location and station, as well as the then ruling kings.

Having gathered such information, and considering the opportunity to compose this book a personal challenge, I could no longer excuse myself from being at your service in regard to what you are requesting and desiring. And so I consigned everything to writing and dispatched it to you—may you be pleased with it, and may God guide you on the right path and grant you success! Already your Creator has bestowed upon you a gift from above, through which He separates you from those who are possessed of mean and murky ambitions.[7] It is as Christ—peace be upon him—said in the pure *Gospel*: "Every gift a person is given by the Divine Spirit comes down from the Gate of Light high above".[8] So be grateful to God for what He gives, praise Him for His gift, and beseech Him to augment His grace—for aid is from Him and through Him, who has no companion!

﴾٤﴿ And now, O noble Sire, [man] of good Umayyad and Qurayshite stock, scion of caliphs, descendant of imams heralding the true religion, now we will

---

350/961–366/976). For the Latin *editio princeps* of Orosius' original work see OrHis; for two editions of the Arabic translation see OrTa' and OrKit (the latter is quoted in our present book); for two important studies on the history and character of this Arabic translation see DaiOr and SahOr *passim*.

5 Eusebius Sophronius Hieronymus, also known as Saint Jerome (Arabic *Yirūnim*, d. 420 CE), a Roman priest and historian from Stridon in Dalmatia, is the author of a universal history titled *Chronicum*, itself an augmented Latin translation of Eusebius of Caesarea's (d. 339 CE) *Κανὼν χρονικός* (book 2 of *Παντοδαπὴ ἱστορία* [lost in Greek]); nothing is known about the Arabic translation of Jerome's *Chronicle* which served Ibn Juljul as a source, and to which he refers here by the transliterated title *al-Qurūniqa*. For a critical edition of Jerome's work see HieCh.

6 It is not obvious what Ibn Juljul means by 'reports' (*akhbār*)—his phrasing *ra'aytuhā* "which I have seen" clearly suggests written (rather than oral) sources, and we will have occasion to observe that at least for some of the relevant material he must have relied on Arabic versions of Greek *gnomologia*.

7 It would appear that this "gift already bestowed from above" refers to the addressee's privilege of birth and nobility of character.

8 This is an abbreviated variation or curtailed paraphrase, not of a passage from the *Gospel* but from the *Epistle of James*, where one reads (1:17): "Every good gift and every perfect gift is from above, and cometh down from the Father of Lights, with whom is no variableness, neither shadow of turning" (21st century King James version); in today's Arabic bible, the passage runs as follows: *kull ʿaṭiyya ṣāliḥa wa-kull mawhiba tāmma hiya min fawq nāzila min ʿinda abī l-anwār alladhī laysa ʿindahū taghyīr wa-lā ẓill dawarān*. The Arabic bible which Ibn Juljul had at his disposal almost certainly offered a different reading, and was based probably on Saint Jerome's Latin translation/revision (completed in 405 CE); on a sidenote, it is quite possible that in Ibn Juljul's quotation the word *bāb* "gate" represents a clerical error for *āb* "father". But why, in a work clearly addressed to an Arab Muslim, quote the *Bible* at all?

begin, with God's help, to lay out what you seek and to set forth what you desire—may God support us in this [task]!

﴾٥﴿ Account of the **first** eminent **generation**: those who spoke about medical wisdom and celestial philosophy

In the *Book of the Thousands*, Abū Maʿshar al-Balkhī the astrologer[9] says: "There are three Hermeses.[10] The first of them is the

1 Hermes[11]

who lived before the Flood. The signification 'Hermes' is a title, just as one says 'Caesar' or 'Khosrow'. In their biographies, the Persians call him Abanjhān.[12] He is the one whose wisdom the Ḥarrānians invoke. [The Persians][13] state that his grandfather was Jayūmart, which is Adam,[14] and the Hebrews state that he is Enoch, which in Arabic is Idrīs".[15]

Abū Maʿshar [further] says: "He was the first to speak about celestial matters, such as stellar motions, and his grandfather Jayūmart taught him the hours of the night and the day. He was the first to build ﴾٦﴿ temples and to glorify God in them. He was the first to investigate medicine and to speak about it. He composed for his contemporaries rhythmic odes and prominent verses

---

9 On Abū Maʿshar and his *Thousands* see note 3 above.

10 In a fairly recent monographic study titled *The Arabic Hermes*, Kevin van Bladel has explored, in magnificent detail, the multifarious origin of the legends surrounding the three Hermeses, and there is no need to reiterate here the findings of his learned travails (BlaAH 121–163)—the more inquisitive reader is encouraged to resort to van Bladel's readily available publication, and to consult moreover the parallel passages in IAU 3.1/41 ff. Suffice it to repeat that Ibn Juljul's account of the three Hermeses represents the earliest extant in Arabic literature, as his explicitly named source, Abū Maʿshar's *Thousands*, is now largely lost.

11 Arabic *Hirmis* < *Ἑρμῆς (ὁ Τρισμέγιστος)*.

12 Abanjhān < Persian Vīvanjhān, the presumed father of the mythical Iranian king Jamshīd, see JuNB 374a and SkJam *passim*; further JulṬab 6 f. note 4 and PinTAM 14 f. The reading *'bnjhdh* is to be emended accordingly.

13 Added from the parallel passage IAU 2.1/45.

14 Jayūmart < Persian Gayōmart, the protoplast of man and the first king in Iranian mythical history, who in Islamic literature is often associated with Adam, see ShaGa *passim*.

15 Idrīs is generally associated in Islamic literature with the biblical patriarch Enoch (Arabic *Khunūkh*); in the *Koran* (19:56), he is called a prophet (*nabiyy*).

on terrestrial and celestial matters. He was the first to warn of the Flood, and he saw that a heavenly disaster would overwhelm the earth with water or fire. His chosen home was Upper Egypt, where he built the pyramids and cities of clay. He feared that knowledge would disappear with the Flood, and so he built monumental temples—there is a mountain in Akhmim known as *birbā*,[16] which he hollowed out, representing in it all the crafts and their applications in the form of lithoglyphs, [drawing] pictures of all the instruments of the craftsmen, and indicating the properties of the sciences through illustrations, because he was driven by a desire to perpetuate these skills for posterity, and because he feared that all trace of it might vanish from the world".

Reports transmitted on the authority of early Muslims confirm that Idrīs was the first to study books and to investigate the sciences; that God revealed to him thirty scrolls; and that he was the first to sew clothes and to wear them. God raised him to a high station.[17]

Abū Maʿshar [also] tells some absurd stories about him, but I have reproduced here only the most true[18] and most plausible. Success is with God the Sublime.

﴾٨﴿ 2
The second Hermes

"[He] belonged to the people of Babylon, residing in this city of the Chaldeans. He lived after the Flood, in the time of Nbryzbāny,[19] who was the first to build [in] the city of Babylon after Nimrod son of Kush.[20] ﴾٩﴿ He was skilled in the knowledge of medicine and philosophy, and acquainted with the inherent properties of numbers. Pythagoras the arithmetician was his pupil.[21] This

16 *birbā* < Coptic ∗*pꜣ-rꜣ-pr*∗ "temple", see DalMM 50—hence the "hollowed-out mountain (*jabal*)" in Akhmim is a metaphor for its imposing temple; earlier on, Ibn Juljul employed the plural *barābī*, which I translated accordingly as "monumental temples".

17 The final sentence of this short paragraph is a quote from the *Koran* (19:57). For passages parallel to the "reports of early Muslims (*salaf*)" see e.g. ReReEn 293 f.

18 Read *bi-aḥaqqahā* (instead of *bi-akhaffahā*).

19 Perhaps read نبوقدناصر (instead of نبريزباني), that is Nebuchadnezzar II, king of the Neo-Babylonian Empire (reg. 605–562 BCE), who is known for his ambitious construction projects in the capital city of Babylon, and also, according to some, associated with building the Hanging Gardens.

20 Nimrod son of Kush (Arabic *Nimrūdh ibn Kūsh*) is a legendary figure; according to *Genesis* 10:8–12, he was king of Babylon and other cities in southern Mesopotamia before he started to build cities like Nineveh in the north.

21 Read *al-arithmāṭīqī* (instead of *al-aritmāṭīqī*) and *tilmīdhahū* (instead of *tilmīdh*). The

Hermes restored the knowledge of medicine, philosophy and mathematics that was obliterated by the Flood of Babylon"—this is what Abū Maʿshar relates.

The aforesaid city of the Chaldeans was the city of the philosophers of the eastern people; their philosophers were the first to set up boundaries and to establish codes of law; they are the philosophers [who influenced] the Persian intellectuals.

﴿١٠﴾ 3
The third Hermes

He resided in the city of Egypt[22] and lived after the Flood. He is the author of the *Book on Venomous Animals*.[23] He was a philosopher and a physician, knowledgeable about the natures of lethal drugs and hostile animals. He travelled and wandered in [different] countries; he knew the foundations and the character of cities, and the mentality of their inhabitants. He spoke well and worthily about the art of alchemy, dealing with various crafts such as [the making of] glass, [the mining of] gems, [the glazing of] earthen vessels, and things like that. He had a pupil whose name is known to be Asclepius.[24] There are some absurd reports and many [other] tales about him—we will [continue to] seek out the ones that are true from among the material found in respectable books, God willing.

﴿١١﴾ 4
Asclepius[25]

This is the pupil of Hermes the Egyptian.[26] His home was the land of the northern regions.[27] Galen, in a book which he composed [and titled] *Exhortation to*

---

connection established here between Hermes and Pythagoras (of Samos, Arabic *Fīthāghūras*, d. ca. 495 BCE) is of course fictitious.

22 It is not clear which ancient Egyptian city Ibn Juljul refers to here—perhaps Heliopolis, but this is just a guess.

23 *Kitāb al-Ḥayawān dhawāt al-sumūm* (pseudepigraphic).

24 For Asclepius see biography 4 below.

25 Arabic *Asqalābiyūs* < Ἀσκληπιός, the god of medicine in Greek mythology.

26 For Hermes 'the Egyptian' see biography 3 above.

27 The term *al-shāmāt* generally denotes the regions north of the Arabian Peninsula, and in particular Greater Syria and Anatolia; it is a plural of *al-shāma*, which literally means "the left" but also, for a people whose primary orientation is directed towards sunrise, "the North". The geographer Yāqūt al-Rūmī (d. 626/1229), having offered a number of fanciful etymological explanations of the term, says that it covers an area which stretches from the Euphrates to the borderlands of Egypt, and from the Syrian desert to the 'Greek Sea' (i.e.

Medicine, mentions that God intimated to [Asclepius]: "Verily,[28] I myself should more fittingly call you an angel rather than call you a man".[29]

Hippocrates, in his book [titled] *The Oaths and Covenant*,[30] mentions that this name, I mean Asclepius, is derived from 'splendour' and 'light' in the language of the Greeks,[31] and that medicine is the craft of Asclepius; [further] that only those may concern themselves with it who lead the same life as Asclepius

---

the Eastern Mediterranean), see YāBul 5/218 f. Ibn Juljul, too, seems to have understood the term in its widest possible sense: thus, speaking about the physician Hippocrates, he equates the Greek island of Cos with the Syrian city of Homs in *al-shāmāt*, cf. the beginning of biography 6 below; another time, speaking about the Athenian philosopher Socrates, he maintains that the latter was a Greek inhabitant of *al-shāmāt*, cf. the beginning of biography 10 below; in a similar vein, the botanist Dioscorides of Anazarbos is described as an Anatolian (*shāmī*) Greek, cf. the beginning of biography 7 below. Ibn Juljul's idiosyncratic employment of the term *al-shām* and its derivations appears to be due partly to his own somewhat shaky grasp of the geography of the Islamic East, and partly to the ambiguity inherent in the term itself.

28 Read *innaka* (instead of *annaka*).

29 The Galenic treatise referred to here is the variously titled *Προτρεπτικὸς ἐπ' ἰατρικήν*, see FiCG 7 f. no. 1 for editions and translations of the Greek text; an Arabic translation, titled *al-Ḥathth ʿalā taʿallum al-ṭibb*, was made in Iraq around the middle of the 3rd/9th century by Ḥubaysh al-Aʿsam, see BergGÜ 37 f. no. 110. In the extant Greek version, only the first, introductory part of the work is preserved, see BarGal 49 f.; the old Arabic translation, too, was based on "a single part/treatise" (*maqāla wāḥida*, see BergGÜ ٤٦ = 37, ult.), but it is not clear how exactly this description should be interpreted; a summary (?) of the first part of Galen's work appears to be preserved in the unique Arabic manuscript Cairo *Taymūr* (akhlāq) 290, see GaS 3/138 no. 151 with BarGal 77 f. There is no doubt that Ibn Juljul possessed an Arabic translation of Galen's *Προτρεπτικός*, but, on the background of the aforesaid findings, it is impossible to even guess at the form, quality or scope of this translation, which brings us finally to the 'divine intimation' that Ibn Juljul apparently extracted from the text. The extant Greek version mentions Asclepius twice (BarGal 114,14 and 132,18), but neither passage can be reconciled easily with Ibn Juljul's quotation—perhaps he radically paraphrased the latter-named passage, which says that "Asclepius and Dionysus, whether they were originally men or born as gods, must be considered worthy of [divine] honours, the one because he discovered medicine, the other because he taught viticulture". However, this statement is quite far removed from Ibn Juljul's wording, and therefore the possibility remains that his 'quotation' might reflect a corresponding passage in the *lost* part of Galen's treatise.

30 This is a reference to the so-called 'Hippocratic Oath' (*Ὅρκος*, Arabic *al-Aymān* "The Oaths" or [!] *al-ʿAhd* "The Covenant"), see FiCH 23 f. no. 14 for editions and translations of the Greek text; the Arabs were generally working with a translation of pseudo-Galen's commentary on the *Ὅρκος*, which was made by Ḥubaysh al-Aʿsam, see BergGÜ 32 no. 87; the full Arabic version of the oath is preserved IAU 3.1/66 f.

31 The etymology of the name Asclepius is not clear—the explanation given by the Arabs may somehow be connected to the term *αἴγλη* "light, splendour"; for a more detailed discussion of the problem see IAU 3.1/37 note 12 and the literature quoted there (esp. RoAC).

in terms of purity, modesty and piety, and that it must not be taught to the wicked nor to the vicious souls—only the noble and the divine, meaning those who recognize the lofty, praiseworthy and sublime Deity,[32] may study it; and that he who is equipped with the knowledge of medicine should be compassionate, virtuous and eager to help people.[33]

In this very book, Hippocrates [also] mentions that [Asclepius] was lifted into the air in a shaft of light.[34]

Galen, in the first treatise of his book [titled] *To Glaucon* the philosopher, remarks: "If only I could be like Asclepius!"[35] And at the beginning of the book [titled] *The Method of Healing*, Galen says: "Ordinary people become convinced[36] of the validity of medicine when they see the divine healing [that happens] in the Temple of Asclepius".[37] Now, this Temple of Asclepius—according to what Orosius the author of *The Histories* relates[38]—was a shrine in the city of Rome, housing an effigy that spoke to people when they asked questions; and that it was Asclepius who, in the days of yore, designed the effigy. The pagans

---

32 Note that for strictly monotheistic reasons, *Ilāh* (not *Allāh*) is used to translate *Θεός*.

33 Asclepius is invoked at the beginning of the Greek 'Hippocratic Oath' together with Apollon, Hygieia and Panacea; in the Arabic version(s), he is invoked next to God (*Allāh*). The bulk of this passage, however, represents a shortened paraphrase obtained, not from the *Ὅρκος* but from the pseudo-Hippocratic *Ποδαπὸν δεῖ εἶναι τὸν ἰατρόν* "How the Physician should be" (Arabic *Tartīb al-ṭibb* "The Etiquette of Medicine" or *al-Waṣiyya* "The Testament" [< *Διαθήκη*])—for the Greek text see SidTH 198ff., for a full Arabic version see IAU 3.1/68; cf. further FiCH 80 no. 171.

34 Hippocrates says no such thing—the present statement reflects a monotheistic re-interpretation and elaboration of the 'divinity' of Asclepius, whom Christian and Muslim commentators allowed to have been taken by God to Himself in this way, cf. IAU 3.1/38 with note 22.

35 Galen's *Πρὸς Γλαύκωνα θεραπευτικά* had been translated into Arabic under the title *Ilā Ighlawqun (fī l-taʾattī li-shifāʾ al-amrāḍ)* by Ḥunayn ibn Isḥāq, see BergGÜ 5f. no. 6; for Greek and Arabic editions see FiCG 58f. no. 70. The above 'quotation', however, is not found in this work, but rather in Galen's *Θεραπευτικὴ μέθοδος* or "The Method of Healing" (Arabic *Ḥīlat al-burʾ*), which Ibn Juljul quotes straight after (where to read *ḥīla* instead of *ḥlya*, a printing error). An Arabic translation of the latter text was made by Ḥubaysh al-Aʿsam, see BergGÜ 13ff. no. 20; a new Greek and a first-time Arabic edition are apparently in preparation, see FiCG 56ff. no. 69. In Kühn's old edition, the underlying Galenic statement, in its proper context, is translated as follows: "Hi vero unam esse omnium curationem existimant; ego contra, si cujusque privatim naturam explorare ad unguem scirem, *utique qualem fuisse Aesculapium mente concipio*, talem me esse putarem; *sed quoniam id fieri non potest*", see GOO 10/206f.

36 Read *yaḥuththu* (instead of *yajibu*).

37 This 'quotation' is not traceable to Galen's *Θεραπευτικὴ μέθοδος* (on which see note 35 above), nor indeed to any other of his writings.

38 On Orosius and his *Histories* cf. note 4 above.

of Rome believed that this effigy was ﴾١٢﴿ constructed in synchrony with the stellar motions, and that it contained [at any given time] the spiritual essence of one [or another] of the seven planets—before Christianity, the religion of the inhabitants of Rome was star-worship. So relates Orosius.[39] He also tells some absurd stories, but we have summoned here only the most plausible to the mind and omitted the ones that are too far-fetched.[40]

Plato, in his book known as *The Laws*,[41] says: "Asclepius was busy worshipping in his temple when a man and a woman approached him for his counsel about a baby that she carried in her belly. Asclepius said to her: 'O sinner! Whilst your husband was in the temple of the Sun-worshippers,[42] praying for your life and lasting welfare, a young man from the tribe of so-and-so had sexual intercourse with you! In three [days time], you will give birth to a malformed creature'—and she did in fact deliver a baby that had two hands [attached] to its chest. There Asclepius affectionately turned to the man and said: 'Listen! You tied the knot with this woman on false assumptions, and so you reaped from her more than you have sown!'"

In the same book, Plato relates that a man, having hidden away some of his money, said to Asclepius: "O Light of the Hearts! I lost my money, can you find it for me?" And Asclepius went with him to his house, where indeed he found it for him. Then he said to the man: "It is only fair that someone who fools around with the blessings of God should be deprived of them. You will lose this money, and it will not return!"—and so it was.

39 Orosius, in his *Histories*, mentions twice the Temple (Latin *templum* > Arabic *bayt* lit. "house" or *miḥrāb al-wathan* "sanctum of the idol") and once the effigy (Latin *lapis* "stone [figure]" > Arabic *ṣūra* "image") of Asclepius—for the original Latin text see OrHis 90, 139 and 192; for an Arabic translation see OrKit 191, 252 and 306. The source of Ibn Juljul's above account remains obscure. Llavero Ruiz, with regard to the 'seven planets', elaborates: "El mundo, antiguamente, estaba dividido en siete regiones, y la gente de cada región adoraba a uno de los siete astros del sistema, ofreciéndoles sacrificios e inmolándoles víctimas, pues creían que sus espíritus les protegían. Estos astros son el Sol, Mercurio, Venus, La Tierra, Marte, Júpiter y Saturno, conocidos por las dos estrellas y los cinco planetas", see ŶulGen 110f. note 17.

40 It is not clear which other stories Ibn Juljul refers to here—as can be seen from the preceding note, Orosius hardly says anything at all about Asclepius.

41 This is a reference, not to Plato's *Νόμοι* but to a pseudo-Platonic magical treatise also titled *al-Nawāmīs* "The Laws" (an araboform plural of *νόμος*). The latter Arabic writing, composed probably between 850 and 900 CE by an unknown author, is today almost entirely lost, and only preserved in a 12th-century CE Latin translation, see HaPAL 52–58.

42 Read *ʿabīd* (instead of *ʿīd*).

[Also] in this book, Plato tells the strange story of a delegation which the king Marinus had sent to Asclepius: whilst the delegates were still with him, he announced the death of Marinus; then they left [and returned home], where indeed they found him dead.[43]

Hippocrates, in his book [titled] *The Oaths*, mentions that the Staff of Asclepius was [taken] from the marshmallow tree, and that the image of a serpent was carved all around it.[44]

Galen says: "He chose a marshmallow stick because he cared for equability—as the marshmallow tree is balanced in terms of [inherent] heat and coldness, and as he heeded the middle ground in all his affairs, he could not but choose a stick from an equable tree; and he carved a serpent around it because this is the longest-living animal, which for him symbolized knowledge that does neither fade nor perish".[45]

Such are the credible accounts that I managed to find on Asclepius in written sources; there are [also] some absurd tales about him in ﴾١٣﴿ the annals of the Christians,[46] not worthy of being [included] in our book. The above testimonies of Hippocrates, Galen and Plato, if indeed they are true, clearly imply that the study of medicine and philosophy was triggered by way of divine revelation and inspiration. And how else could it have been, judging from the preceding reports?[47]

---

43 The full, rather long version of this story is found IAU 3.1/309–312. The identity of Marinus (Arabic *Mārīnūs*) is obscure—the geographer-historian al-Masʿūdī (d. 345/956) registers a certain *Mār(i)nūs* among the ancient kings of Babylonia (MasMur 2/97, ult.), whilst Shlomo Pines equates the name with *Μίνως*, the mythical king of Crete (PiQuo 236–239).

44 This statement is not found in Hippocrates' *Ὅρκος*, nor in the extant Arabic version of the oath; cf. note 30 above.

45 This short paragraph radically condenses and slightly modifies certain observations made in the pseudo-Galenic "Commentary on the Covenant of Hippocrates" (**Εἰς τὸ Ἱπποκράτους περὶ ὅρκου**, Arabic *Tafsīr ʿAhd Buqrāṭ*)—an edition of the Greek text is in preparation, see FiCG 141f. no. 390; parts of the old Arabic translation by Ḥubaysh al-Aʿsam, including his uncle Ḥunayn's super-commentary, are preserved IAU 3.1/45–52 = RoAC 64–76 (where both the marshmallow and the serpent are dealt with at greater length).

46 Orosius' *Histories* (cf. note 4 above), Jerome's *Chronicle* (cf. note 5 above), Isidore of Seville's *Origins* (cf. note 159 below), and perhaps others.

47 The 'preceding reports' are likely to refer back to the *entire* biographical material presented so far in Ibn Juljul's book.

﴾١٥﴿ 5
Apollon[48]

One also says ‘Apollo’.[49] He was the first sage in the land of the Romans and Greeks to speak about medicine. He invented the letters of the Greek alphabet[50] for the king Amenophis.[51] He [not only] spoke about medicine [but also] developed it rationally and practised it. He lived after Moses—peace be upon him—in the time of Barak the judge.[52] I have seen glorious [as well as] absurd recollections of him, but in regard to his many miraculous deeds he is up there with Asclepius.[53]

﴾١٦﴿ The **second generation:**
ancient Greek sages who spoke about and excelled at medicine and philosophy

The first of them is

6
Hippocrates[54]

the eminent, who hailed from the tribe of Asclepius.[55] His home was the city of Cos, which is the city of Homs in the land of the northern regions.[56]

He is the one who [not only] spoke about medicine [but also] wrote important treatises and [other] works on that [subject]—thus, he authored the books [titled] *Aphorisms, Prognostic, Epidemics, Acute Diseases, Bone Setting and Dislocation, The Nature of Man, Humours, Ulcers, Head Injuries, Waters and Airs*, as well as many others.[57]

---

48 Arabic *Abūlun* < *Ἀπόλλων*, a central and highly complex Greek deity.

49 Arabic *Abulluh*, which reflects the Latin form of the Greek name.

50 Literally “writing” (*kitāb*).

51 Amenophis (Arabic *Mināfis*) is the Greek form of Amenhotep, the name of several Egyptian pharaohs, princes and noblemen.

52 For the story of Barak the judge (Arabic *Barāq al-ḥākim*) see *Judges* 4–5.

53 For Asclepius see biography 4 above.

54 Arabic *Buqrāṭ* < *Ἱπποκράτης*, the famous Greek physician (d. ca. 370 BCE).

55 For Asclepius see biography 4 above; the ‘tribe’ (*ahl*) of Asclepius are the Greeks.

56 There are two geographical blunders in this sentence: first, Cos (Arabic *Qū* < *Κῶ*, genitive [!] of *Κῶς*) is an island in the Aegean Sea, not a ‘city’ (*madīna*); and second, it is in any case not identical with the Syrian city of Homs (Emesa). On the term *al-shāmāt* “the northern regions” cf. note 27 above.

57 This highly eclectic list of Hippocratic writings includes (in the given order): *Ἀφορισμοί* >

He was an excellent [man], devout and ascetic, who treated illness with circumspection. He roamed and wandered about in [many] countries. The pupil who succeeded him [as a physician] for the inhabitants of his city[58] was Polybus.[59] [Hippocrates] lived during the reign of Ardashir[60] Bahman ﴿١٧﴾ the Persian, grandfather of Dārā son of Dārā.[61] Galen, in an epistle whose [title] translates as[62] *The Physician should be a Philosopher*,[63] mentions that[64] Ardashir Bahman sent for Hippocrates to cure him from an illness he had contracted, and that Hippocrates refused to oblige because Ardashir was an enemy of the Greeks. [Galen also says] that when two Greek kings called upon him to treat them, he complied because they led a decent life, but he did not agree to stay with them after they had recovered from their illness. [Further] that Ardashir, in order to gain Hippocrates' companionship, offered him one thousand *qinṭār* of gold,[65] and that Hippocrates declined.[66]

---

al-Fuṣūl (FiCH 21ff. no. 13), *Προγνωστικόν > Taqdimat al-maʿrifa* (FiCH 10f. no. 3), *Ἐπιδημίαι > Afīdhīmiyā* (FiCH 12–17 nos 6–7 and 26–36 nos 16–20), *Περὶ διαίτης ὀξέων > [Tadbīr] al-amrāḍ al-ḥādda* (FiCH 11f. no. 4), *Μοχλικός* and/or *Περὶ ἀγμῶν > al-Jabr wa-l-khalʿ* (FiCH 21 no. 12), *Περὶ φύσιος ἀνθρώπου > Ṭabīʿat al-insān* (FiCH 39f. no. 25 with 18f. no. 10), *Περὶ χυμῶν > al-Akhlāṭ* (FiCH 36f. no. 21), *Περὶ ἑλκῶν > al-Qurūḥ* (FiCH 44 no. 33), *Περὶ τῶν ἐν κεφαλῇ τρωμάτων > Jirāḥāt al-ra's* (FiCH 18 no. 8), *Περὶ ἀέρων ὑδάτων τόπων > al-Miyāh wa-l-ahwiya [wa-l-buldān]* (FiCH 7–10 no. 2). These (and other) Hippocratic works, which reached the Arabs mainly through translations of *Galenic commentaries*, would at least in theory have been available to Ibn Juljul, cf. BergGÜ 32–36 nos 88–96, 99 and 102.

58 Meaning the island of Cos, cf. note 56 above.

59 Read *Fūlūbus* < *Πόλυβος* (instead of *Fūlūniyus*). Polybus (fl. ca. 400 BCE), also a native of Cos, was Hippocrates' student and son-in-law. Ibn Juljul's transliteration *Fūlūniyus* may be due to a confusion with the name of Polybus' father, a certain Apollonius.

60 Read, here and in what follows, *Ardashīr* (instead of *Azdashīr*, a simple [clerical?] error).

61 On Ardashir Bahman, his son Dārā I and his grandson Dārā II—members of the *legendary* Kayanid dynasty of Iranian kings that are said to have ruled before the Achaemenids—see KMBah and TafDā *passim*; Ardashir Bahman is sometimes identified with Artaxerxes I by Arab (and modern!) authors, e.g. ŶulGen 111 note 24. Cf. also note 66 below.

62 Read *tarjamatuhā* (instead of *tarjamahā*).

63 This is a reference to Galen's *Ὅτι ὁ ἄριστος ἰατρὸς καὶ φιλόσοφος*, which had been translated into Arabic by Ḥunayn ibn Isḥāq and, again, by ʿĪsā ibn Yaḥyā under the (full) title *Fī Anna l-ṭabīb al-fāḍil faylasūf* "That the Best Physician is a Philosopher", see BergGÜ 36 no. 103 and FiCG 9f. no. 3.

64 Read *anna* (instead of *inna*).

65 *qinṭār* is a weight which, when used for a large amount of gold, equals 42.33 kg, see HiMW 35f.; 1000 *qinṭār* would accordingly add up to the astronomical sum of roughly 40 tons (!).

66 The short anecdotes recounted here by Ibn Juljul on the authority of Galen are pale reflections of certain statements which the latter makes in his aforesaid 'epistle' (*risāla*), often invoking Hippocrates—to wit (in the translation of Daremberg): "Pourrions-nous, à notre

In the same treatise, Galen [moreover] says: "He who seeks the science of Hippocrates must follow his example in terms of excellence, [he must] desire virtue and shun vice".[67]

I have seen a charming story about Hippocrates, the gist of which I will recount [here] in order to illustrate his excellence. Polemon,[68] the author of *The Physiognomy*,[69] claimed in this book that he could infer the character of a person[70] from his appearance. [When] the students of Hippocrates got together, one of them said to his fellows: "Do you know of anybody in our present age who is better than Hippocrates, this exceptional man?" Some answered: "We do not", but one of them said: "Let us go and check out the matter with the science of Polemon and his claims about physiognomy!" And so they drew a picture of Hippocrates, took it to Polemon, and said to him: "O man of distinction! Look at this person and pass a judgement on his character based on appearance". [Polemon] inspected the figure, assessed its body parts in relation to each other, and then gave a verdict, saying: "This is a man who likes fornication". The students replied: "Liar! This is a picture of Hippocrates the sage", but [Polemon] said to them: "There is no doubt that my science speaks the truth—[go] ask him, the man has no interest in lying". So they returned to [see] Hippocrates, and when they told him the affair, what they had done and what Polemon had

---

époque, citer un homme si détaché de l'argent, qu'il se contente de celui que réclament les besoins indispensables du corps? Trouverait-on un homme qui pourrait non-seulement enseigner par ses discours, mais démontrer par la pratique, que la limite naturelle de la richesse est de n'avoir ni faim, ni soif, ni froid? S'il se trouve un tel médecin, il dédaignera les faveurs d'Artaxerce [!] et de Perdiccas; jamais il ne paraîtra devant le premier; quant au second, il le traitera s'il souffre de quelque maladie qui réclame l'art d'Hippocrate; mais il ne se croira pas obligé de rester toujours auprès de lui, et se rendra à Cranon, à Thasos et dans d'autres bourgades, pour y soigner les pauvres", see DarOG 1/5; for the Greek text see GOO 1/57 f.; for an Arabic edition with German translation of Galen's epistle see BaGal.

67 This appears to be another summarizing paraphrase of certain Galenic observations, such as (in the translation of Daremberg): "Comment aimerait-il le travail celui qui s'enivre, qui se gorge d'aliments et se livre aux plaisirs de Vénus, qui, pour le dire en un mot, est l'esclave de son ventre et de ses penchants lubriques. Il demeure donc établi que le vrai médecin est l'ami de la tempérance, et qu'il est en même temps le disciple de la vérité", see DarOG 1/6; for the Greek text see GOO 1/59; cf. further BaGal.

68 Arabic *Iflīmūn* < *Πολέμων*, that is Marcus Antonius *Polemon* of Laodicea, an Anatolian Greek aristocrat, politician and intellectual (d. ca. 144 CE, not "vivió en el siglo III d.C." [ŶulGen 111 note 25]).

69 On Polemon's *Physiognomy* (*Φυσιογνωμονία*, Arabic *al-Firāsa*) and its Greek, Latin and Arabic manifestations see SFSS *passim*.

70 Read *al-insān* (instead of *al-asnān*).

said, he replied: "Polemon is right—I like fornication, but I restrain myself". This [story] illustrates the excellence of Hippocrates, his self-control, and [how] he trained his soul to be virtuous.[71]

In his book [titled] *The Covenant and Oaths*, [Hippocrates] advocates that no one should study medicine unless he belongs to those people who are modest, righteous, and compassionate towards their fellow human beings; [further] that he should be handsome, neatly dressed, trained in the four basic sciences,[72] judicious, respectable, and intelligent.[73]

﴿٢١﴾ 7
Dioscorides[74]

[He was] a native of Anazarbos,[75] an Anatolian[76] Greek botanist who lived after Hippocrates. He interpreted the majority of Hippocrates' writings,[77] and

---

71 It is clear that this story is chronologically incoherent, as Hippocrates and Polemon are separated by almost 500 years. In Greek literature, the protagonists are Socrates the philosopher and Zopyrus the physiognomist; it seems certain that Ibn Juljul's Hippocrates is a misreading of Socrates (Arabic بقراط for the former, سقراط for the latter), and it is likely that he (or his source) replaced Zopyrus by Polemon who, among the Arabs, was the most well-known 'ancient' physiognomist. In Arabic gnomological literature, the story reappears in a much shorter form, running as follows: "A man who professed [to be an expert in] physiognomy, having been shown a picture of Socrates, said: 'This is someone who is dominated by a desire for depravity'. [Hearing] this the people laughed and said: 'This is Socrates, the most decent of men!' But Socrates said to them: 'Wait! The man does not lie. By nature, I am as he said, except that I control myself and vanquish my desire'". For the gnomologium and its literary context see GuGWL 110 f. no. 48 with 326 f.; for a much longer and more intricate Arabic version of Ibn Juljul's story, also featuring Hippocrates and Polemon, cf. the introductory part of the so-called 'Istanbul Polemon', which has been edited and translated by Antonella Ghersetti in SFSS 465–485 (the story on 468–475).

72 On the "four basic sciences" (*al-mihan al-arba'*) see the following note.

73 This passage, though explicitly linked to the so-called 'Hippocratic Oath' (cf. note 30 above), represents a paraphrased excerpt from the short pseudo-Hippocratic *Testament* (cf. note 33 above), for which see SidTH 201. The "four basic sciences" (*al-mihan al-arba'*) are the mathematical, natural, theological and logical sciences, see MPC 77 (English) = ٧٨ (Arabic); the (reconstructed) Greek version of the *Testament*, if indeed it reflects Ibn Juljul's source, speaks of *γραμματική*, *ἀστρονομία/γεωμετρία*, *μουσική* and *φιλοσοφία*, see SidTH 198 § 3.

74 Arabic *Diyāsqūrīdūs* < *Διοσκουρίδης*, the famous Greek botanist (d. ca. 90 CE).

75 Anazarbos (Ἀνάζαρβος) was an ancient city in Cilicia; its Arabic name *'Ayn Zarba* is a (partly arabicized) transliteration of the variant Greek form *Ἀνάζαρβα*.

76 On the connotations surrounding the term *shāmī*, here translated "Anatolian", cf. note 27 above.

77 This is a strange and factually untenable statement on the part of Ibn Juljul, especially as

he is the most knowledgeable among those who spoke about the very principle of medical treatment. He is the chief authority on simple drugs, [which] he discussed according to types and categories, without speaking of [humoral] degrees. He authored a work [titled] *The Five Treatises*,[78] which is something nobody before him had accomplished in the manner he did.

Galen says: "I have studied fourteen books on simple drugs, [written] by different people, but I have never seen anything more perfect on this [subject] than the work of Dioscorides, the native of Anazarbos".[79] All those who came after him followed the example [given] in this [work], through which he immortalized useful knowledge and [laid down] a comprehensive foundation. The meaning of his name in Greek is "God's herbalist", because the word *diyāshqūr* [signifies] "herbalist" and *diyūs* [denotes] "God"—it is as though the designation "God's herbalist" is another way of saying 'inspired by God to talk about trees and herb[s]'.[80]

He [also wrote] two treatises on poisons,[81] in which he advances some good stuff.[82]

---

the verb he uses in the present phrase is *tarjama*, lit. "he translated (!)"; the variant *fassara*, lit. "he commented on", obtained from another source (see JulṬab 21 note 2), leaves us with the same problem.

78 This is a paraphrastic reference to Dioscorides' chef-d'œuvre *Περὶ ὕλης ἰατρικῆς* (Latin *De materia medica*), which consists of five books; for the Greek text see DioMM. The work was translated into Arabic, directly from the Greek, by Iṣṭifān ibn Basīl, in Baghdad around the middle of the 3rd/9th century, and had been available in Spain by the end of that century, see UllMM 23; its original Arabic title appears to have been *al-Ḥashā'ish fī hayūlā l-ṭibb*, see UllMed 259. It is worth noting that Ibn Juljul himself, five years prior to the completion of the *Generations*, published a short adjunctive commentary (*tafsīr*) on Dioscorides' *Materia medica*—for an Arabic edition with German translation of this commentary see DietMM; for the rather illustrious history of Dioscorides' work in Arab Spain cf. UllMM 61–64.

79 Putting aside the somewhat random specification 'fourteen', Ibn Juljul here quotes (and slightly abridges) a passage from Galen's *Περὶ κράσεως καὶ δυνάμεως τῶν ἁπλῶν φαρμάκων*, which had been translated into Arabic by Ḥubaysh al-Aʿsam, see BergGÜ 23f. no. 53; in this passage, Galen favourably contrasts Dioscorides with other like-minded writers, saying (in Kühn's translation): "At Anazarbensis Dioscorides quinque libris materiam omnem utilem absolvit [...] Et mihi utique videtur omnium perfectissime tractatum de materia medicamentorum confecisse", see GOO 11/794.

80 These etymological exercises are hard to account for: Ibn Juljul himself knew no Greek, and the source of the information is unclear. 'Dioscorides' means "descending from the sons of Zeus" (*Διόσκουροι* + *-ίδης*), cf. EDG 1/338.

81 The 'correct' plural forms of Arabic *samm* "poison" are *sumūm* or *simām*; the form *samā'im*, which Ibn Juljul strangely employs here, is strictly speaking a plural of *samūm* "hot wind", cf. LaLex 1419a and 1420a.

82 The "two treatises on poisons" refer to the pseudo-Dioscoridic books VI and VII, which

﴿٢٣﴾ 8
Plato[83] the sage

[He was] a native of the city of Athens, an ancient Greek philosopher and physician, someone who understood astronomy and the natures of numbers. He [wrote] a book on medicine which he addressed to his pupil Timaeus,[84] and books, nay, tomes on philosophy. Nobody before him had spoken about the composition [of matter] like he did, who on that [basis] discovered the texture of the [divine] weave[85]—his is a discourse relating ﴿٢٤﴾ to the five compositional proportions, which are the only ones that can be found in all existing composites.[86] Once he had fully grasped the natures of numbers and understood the five compositional proportions, he turned his attention to knowing the world as a whole; he realized the positions of the particles which combine and intermix in [all] their different shades and tints to make a harmonious, proportionate ensemble.[87] This led him to the concept of the Form: he postulated a general movement as the origin of [all] particular movements, then

---

deal with toxicological matters; they bear the titles *Περὶ δηλητηρίων φαρμάκων* (Arabic *Fī l-Sumūm*) and *Περὶ ἰοβόλων* (Arabic *Fī l-Ḥayawān dhawāt al-sumūm*), see UllMed 258 with note 3 and GaS 3/60 nos 2 and 3.

83 Arabic *Aflāṭūn* < *Πλάτων*, the famous Greek philosopher (d. 348–347 BCE).

84 This is clearly a somewhat misconceived reference to Plato's dialogue *Τίμαιος* (Arabic *Ṭīmāwus*), a speculative treatise on physics and the deeper foundations of philosophy. The historicity of Timaeus (the person) is doubtful, for he only appears as a literary character in the eponymous dialogue; he was certainly no 'pupil' (*tilmīdh*) of Plato. The *Timaeus* had been translated into Arabic by Yūḥannā ibn al-Biṭrīq (fl. early 3rd/9th century) and/or, a few decades later, by Ḥunayn ibn Isḥāq, see NadFih 1/246,15 f. Judging from Ibn Juljul's remarks, it seems highly questionable whether he had ever seen this work himself.

85 *dībāj*, here translated "weave", is an arabicized form of Persian *dēbā(h)*, lit. "pannus sericus versicolor; brocade", see VuLex 1/946; for *dībāj* as a potential technical term see the following note.

86 This rather problematic passage has been discussed at some length in IAU 3.1/133 f. note 5, to which the interested reader is encouraged to resort. Suffice it here to repeat that Ibn Juljul's extremely terse (and somewhat garbled) account appears to evoke the so-called Platonic solids, five perfect geometrical shapes consisting of triangles that form the building blocks of all matter: the tetrahedron (corresponding to the element fire), the octahedron (~ air), the icosahedron (~ water), the hexahedron (~ earth), and the dodecahedron (representing the shape into which God moulded the universe as a whole). In this context, the term *dībāj* (cf. the preceding note) may constitute a faint reflection of the Greek verb *διαζωγραφέω*, which in the relevant Platonic passage (*Timaeus* 55c) is used to describe God's "decorating" the universe with the fifth (non-elementary) polyhedron.

87 Here again, the object of comparison is a multicoloured, richly decorated and intricately patterned item of woven fabric (*dībāj*).

he divided these [moving forms] according to [their] numerical proportion[s], and [finally] he interposed the compositional particles. In this way, he arrived at the concept of conceivable forms; the texture of the [divine] weave and the makeup of all its compositional parts became apparent to him, and he [also] wrote a book on it.[88]

He spoke wonderful words about philosophy, and he was one of those who laid down norms and rules for the people of his time—his books [titled] *The Republic* and *The Laws* [testify] to that.[89] [Plato] lived during the reign of Darius 'the Bastard',[90] the father of that Darius who was killed by Alexander[91]—he [thus] lived after Hippocrates, during the reign of Alexander's father Philip,[92] when the Persians held sway over the Greco-Romans.[93]

﴿٢٥﴾ 9
Aristotle[94] the Macedonian

[He hailed] from Macedonia, a region [in the ancestral realm] of the Greek people. [He is] their [chief] philosopher, their orator and their physician, the most knowledgeable, most brilliant and most talented of them all. He did speak about medicine, but his primary field was philosophy, on which he [wrote] poems[95] and works [in prose]. For example: his book [titled] *Lecture on Physics*,

88 The *Timaeus*, in which such subjects are discussed. Llavero Ruiz misunderstood the whole passage, cf. ŶulGen 44.

89 These are references to Plato's *Πολιτεία* (Arabic *al-Siyāsa*) and, respectively, *Νόμοι* (Arabic *al-Nawāmīs* [pluralis fractus of *nāmūs* < *νόμος*]). Both works had become available in Arabic by the middle of the 3rd/9th century, through Ḥunayn ibn Isḥāq's commentary (*Republic*) or translation (*Laws*), see NadFih 1/246,5—it is not altogether clear, however, whether these two works were translated in their entirety; to which extent they may have been based on Galen's summaries; and what, if anything, Ibn Juljul had in front of himself.

90 Arabic *Dārā Naṭū*, that is the Achaemenid king-of-kings Darius II (reg. 423–404 BCE), who is sometimes referred to in Greek sources as *νόθος* (> Arabic *naṭū*) "bastard".

91 Darius 'the Bastard' was the great-grandfather (not the father) of Darius III (reg. 336–330 BCE); *al-Iskandar* < *Ἀλέξανδρος*, that is *Alexander* the Great (d. 323 BCE).

92 Arabic *Filbus* < *Φίλιππος*, that is Philip II of Macedonia (reg. 359–336 BCE).

93 Ibn Juljul here gives two approximate dates for the lifetime of Plato—the first covers his childhood and youth, the second his old age.

94 Arabic *Arisṭāṭālīs* < *Ἀριστοτέλης*, the famous Greek polymath (d. 322 BCE, not "332" [ŶulGen 112 note 35]).

95 Even though Aristotle is less known as a poet, he "composed enough poetry to fill two papyrus rolls in the ancient collections of his works", see FordAP ix and *passim*. However, it is almost certain that none of Aristotle's (mostly lyrical) poems were ever rendered into Arabic, as the patrons of the translation movement, and by extension the translators themselves, had no particular interest in literary or historical Greek works, cf. GuGT 1

in which he deals comprehensively with the five principles that are found [in nature], namely matter, form, place, time and motion; then his books *On General Existence* and *On Particular Existence*; [or] like his book *Celestial Influences*; then his book[s] *On Animals* and *On Plants*; then his book *On Minerals*; in his book *On the Definitions of Logic*—without which there is no way to understand the art of reasoning—he talked about the meanings of speech, the peculiarities of expression with regard to both single [words] and compound [sentences], and the combined effects of such syntactical units when put together with the aim of producing a logical proof; he [authored] books on [many] branches of science, like *The Orators* and *The Poets*, or *The Refutation of Sophistry*; his book about the higher entity, which he named *Macrocosm*, is [also known as] *The Heaven and the Earth*; his book about monotheism he named *Divinity*; and he [left] *Precepts* and *Political Writings*.[96]

﴿٢٦﴾ [Aristotle] was the teacher of Alexander, son of Philip,[97] to whom he [wrote] wonderful letters, like the one he sent when [Alexander] had conquered the land of Persia. [It was that Alexander] dispatched a message to him, saying: "O distinguished master! I found in the land of Persia people possessing sound judgement and sophistication, the likes of whom can be expected to grab the reign. So I am decided to kill them all. Your opinion on this?" Aris-

---

and 139ff. Therefore, Ibn Juljul's reference to "poems" (*ash'ār*) is much more likely to be an allusion to Aristotle's *Poetics* (Περὶ ποιητικῆς, Arabic *Fī l-Shi'r*), presumably in the translation of Abū Bishr Mattā ibn Yūnus (d. 328/940), see NadFih 1/263,27.

96 This paragraph offers a highly selective, at times misconceived (and misconceivable) list of Aristotelian and pseudo-Aristotelian writings. Sticking to the sequence and somewhat idiosyncratic terminology given here by Ibn Juljul, definitive or speculative identifications are as follows: *al-Samāʿ al-ṭabīʿī* (i.q. *Samʿ al-kiyān*) < Φυσικὴ ἀκρόασις; *Fī l-Kawn al-ʿāmm* and *Fī l-Kawn al-khāṣṣ* < Περὶ γενέσεως καὶ φθορᾶς (and presumably others, cf. JulṬab 27 note 5); *al-Āthār al-ʿulwiyya* < Μετεωρολογικά; *Fī l-Ḥayawān* < Περὶ τὰ ζῷα ἱστορίαι / Περὶ ζῴων μορίων / Περὶ ζῴων κινήσεως / Περὶ πορείας ζῴων / Περὶ ζῴων γενέσεως; *Fī l-Nabāt* < Περὶ φυτῶν (pseudo); the work *Fī l-Maʿādin* is a pseudepigraph, unless it refers to certain sections in the *Meteorologica* where the formation of 'fossiles' and metals is discussed; *Fī Ḥudūd al-manṭiq* seems to be a collective reference to books I–V of the so-called Ὄργανον; *al-Khuṭabāʾ* and *al-Shuʿarāʾ* seem to represent the Ῥητορική and, respectively, Περὶ ποιητικῆς; *al-Radd ʿalā l-sūfisṭāʾiyya* (*sic*) < Περὶ σοφιστικῶν ἐλέγχων (book VI of the *Organon*); *al-ʿĀlam al-kabīr* or *al-Samāʾ* (Latin addition *et mundo* > *wa-l-ʿālam*) < Περὶ οὐρανοῦ; *al-Rubūbiyya* (i.q. *Uthūlūjiyā Arisṭū*) < Θεολογία (pseudo); *Waṣāyā* < ∗Παραγγέλματα∗ (pseudo); and *Siyāsāt* < Πολιτικά. For a long, not unrepresentative inventory of 'Aristotelian' writings in the Arabic tradition see e.g. IAU 3.1/172–181 (with the literature quoted there); for Arabic translations of Aristotelian and pseudo-Aristotelian writings, most of which had been accomplished in the course of the 3rd/9th and early 4th/10th centuries, see e.g. AncGS *passim*.

97 Alexander the Great, son of Philip II of Macedonia, cf. notes 91 and 92 above.

totle replied: "You may have decided to kill them all, and you may well have the power to [inflict] this upon them, but you will still not be able to extinguish their country, nor change the air they [breathe] or the water they [drink].[98] Win them over through kindness and thus gain their loyalty! Greetings". Alexander accepted his counsel, did exactly as advised, and the Persians became his most obedient subjects.[99]

[Aristotle wrote] for him an epistle in eight chapters, dealing with the organization of his empire and all its aspects and affairs. This book is [titled] *The Policy of Good Government*, and [also] known as *The Secret of Secrets*[100]—nobody before him had [done anything] like it. Inside, there are the [following] eight sayings which summarize all principles of commonwealth, to wit:

> The *world* is a garden, *government* its fence;
> *government* is power, sheltered by *laws*;
> *laws* are policies, controlled by the *ruler*;
> the *ruler* is a shepherd, supported by the *army*;
> the *army* are helpers, sustained by *capital*;
> *capital* is wealth, gathered by the *subjects*;
> the *subjects* are servants, pacified by *justice*;
> *justice* is the concord that safeguards the *world*.

These are words of political philosophy, each being connected to the one that precedes and explained by the one that follows, with the last [word] linking up to the first. When he was dying, [Aristotle] ordered to be buried under an octagonal tomb, each of whose sides were to be inscribed with one of those eight sayings.

---

98 That is to say: killing the elites is no solution, as the next generation of Persians, brought up in the same environment, would eventually pose the same threat.

99 This story, among many others, is taken from the highly influential, pseudo-Aristotelian writing "The Secret of Secrets" (Arabic *Sirr al-asrār* > Latin *Secretum secretorum*), also known as "The Policy of Good Government" (*al-Siyāsa fī tadbīr al-riyāsa*)—Ibn Juljul himself, in the following paragraph, explicitly cites this work as his source. The *Sirr al-asrār* is most probably a genuine Arabic production (not a translation from Greek), composed in the early 4th/10th century in the Islamic East—in fact, Ibn Juljul's very reference to it constitutes a *terminus ante quem* for its dissemination (cf. also biography **23** below). The Arabic text of the *Sirr al-asrār* is edited in BadUṣ 65–171; a still unmatched study of this work is ManSA.

100 Cf. the preceding note.

﴿٢٧﴾ There is disagreement regarding his death. Some say: "He died when his time had come, and was buried in the usual way"; others say: "He was lifted into the sky in a shaft of light".[101] In the annals of the Greeks it is stated that God intimated to [Aristotle]: "I myself should more fittingly call you an angel rather than call you a man".[102] [The extent of] his sagacious knowledge is too vast to mention.

He [also] authored[103] a book on the confirmation of [...[104]], which is known as *The Apple*.[105]

﴿٣٠﴾ 10
Socrates[106]

[He was] an ancient Greek inhabiting the northern regions.[107] Philosophy, asceticism and pious devotion were his main concerns. He had no interest in writing books. He used to seek shelter in a wine cask, and did not build a house nor settle down. He wrapped himself in a cloak, taking nothing else for himself.[108]

[One day] the king of his part [of the world] happened across him. As he stared at Socrates, and as the latter reproved him for it, the king said: "What an ugly sight you are!" Socrates replied: "This is not up to me. I have achieved all that I possibly could,[109] meaning a nobility of character". The king: "If you

101 Ibn Juljul used almost exactly the same phrase, on the spurious authority of Hippocrates, in his account of Asclepius, cf. biography 4 above.

102 Here again, Ibn Juljul quotes a statement he had reserved, earlier on, for Asclepius, cf. biography 4 above; note that in the present case he refers to 'Greek annals', whilst the same phrase is cited, in the biography of Asclepius, on the authority of Galen.

103 Read *allafahū* (instead of *al-lugha*).

104 *Lacuna*. JulṬab 29 note 45 suggests that the missing words are *baqā' al-nafs* "the immortality of the soul", which would be in line with the topical frame of the writing specified immediately hereafter as *The Apple*.

105 The pseudo-Aristotelian writing "The Apple" (Arabic *al-Tuffāḥa* > Latin *De pomo*) is a 10th century CE neoplatonic production of unknown authorship; it owes its title to the smell of an apple which periodically revitalized the dying Aristotle as he was lecturing on immortality. For an edition of the Latin text with German translation see AMpo.

106 Arabic *Suqrāṭ* < *Σωκράτης*, the famous Greek philosopher (d. 399 BCE).

107 On the term *al-shāmāt* "the northern regions" cf. note 27 above.

108 Although Socrates allegedly was indifferent to material wealth, earthly pleasures and personal comfort, the latter half of this short paragraph, and especially the evocation of a wine cask (*dann*), reflects a narrative confusion with the lifestyle of Diogenes 'the Cynic' of Sinope (d. 323 BCE).

109 Read *tatmīmuhū* (instead of *ttmmymh*, a printing error).

had come to us, we would have given you [things]". Socrates: "What would you have given to me?" [The king]: "Silk, gold, and pearls!" Socrates: "I see you are trying to dazzle me with the spittle of worms, stones from the earth, and foundlings in oyster shells! Much better is to aim for something higher than that!" [And when] the king said to him: "You are one of my slaves", Socrates replied: "And you are the slave of my slave". "How so?" asked the king, and Socrates said: "Because I am a man who dominates his noxious desire[s], whereas you are a man ﴾٣١﴿ who is dominated by his desire[s]—therefore, you are the slave of my slave". [Then] the king said to him: "What made you choose a wine cask to live in?" Socrates replied: "I cut myself off all fugacious burden". The king: "And if the wine cask breaks apart?" Socrates: "If the wine cask breaks apart, the place [on which it rests] does not". At that point the king, refuted, turned away from him.[110]

Later [the king] discussed [Socrates'] case in private with his special advisers, who were into fire- and[111] star-worship. They suggested to him that he kill Socrates, which is what he set out to do. When Socrates got wind of the king's intention, he did not quit [his place], saying: "Death is not a bad but a good thing, for it completes the human condition". And so he was taken and brought [before the king]; seventy elders testified against him, [claiming] that he had denigrated their gods, and he was sentenced to death. To his wife, who was in tears, he said: "What makes you cry?", and as she replied: "You are going to be killed unjustly!", he said: "Would you rather see me killed justly?"[112] Then he was executed.[113] When [the authorities] wanted to kill him, and one of his students said to him: "What are we to do with your corpse, if you die?", he replied: "Whoever needs the room will take care of cleaning it up".[114] Some of his students said to him: "Write your knowledge down for us in books!",

---

110 This paragraph represents a curtailed fusion of two separate, albeit topically related anecdotes that are found abundantly in Arabic gnomological literature, and that are partly influenced by the well-known, probably apocryphal encounter between Diogenes 'the Cynic' and Alexander the Great. For the relevant gnomologia see GuGWL 90 f. no. 10 and 94–97 no. 20 with the detailed commentary on 288–291 and 297 f.; for the 'breaking cask' cf. also ibid. 86 f. no. 6a with 283–286 (where the interlocutor is not a king but a sophist)—Gutas remarks (p. 286) that "in the Arabic tradition, the barrel, the trademark of Diogenes, is transferred to Socrates, through a fusion of the personalities of the two philosophers that originated with the Cynic tradition of Socrates".

111 Read *wa-ʿalā* (instead of *ʿalā*).

112 For this short exchange between Socrates and his wife see the Arabic gnomologium in GuGWL 96 f. no. 23 with 300 ff.

113 Note that there is no mention of hemlock poisoning here.

114 Cf. GuGWL 98 f. no. 24 with 302 ff.

but he replied: "I am not going to entrust knowledge to the skin of sheep!"[115] He used to say to his students: "My dear sons! Conceal behind a veil who you [really] are, if you do not already do so; be wary of the world, if you have not yet adopted this attitude; consider [the world] to be a thorn, and watch where you put your feet; beware of indulging in the pleasures of this world, for the senses of those hearts that are attached to them remain unreceptive to the Almighty".

A man said to him: "O benevolent teacher! What is the hallmark of God?", and he replied: "Speech that is not constrained by ignorance".

A[nother] man said to him: "O teacher! What is the reason for the creation of the world?", and he replied: "The generosity of God".

Socrates often sat with a shoemaker, a man called Simon,[116] whose acquaintance he had made.[117]

Socrates said: "I do not think that the soul knows what it has been promised"; and [when] one of his students said to him: "Can a wise man not [make any such] promise to it?", he replied: "If it knew, it would fly away, to nobody's avail".

We have mentioned Aristotle before Socrates only because of the former's fame and distinction—[in reality] Socrates was the master of Plato, and Plato was the master and teacher of Aristotle.

﴾٣٣﴿ 11
Democritus[118]

[He was] a homeland Greek.[119] Philosophy was his main concern. He was the one who spoke about indivisible particles and who [wrote] books on this [subject], according to his school [of thought].[120] He lived in the days of Socrates.

---

115 Cf. GuGWL 96f. no. 21 with 298f.

116 This is a reference to Simon (Arabic *Shaymūn*) 'the shoemaker' (*Σίμων σκυτοτόμος*), a 'working' philosopher and associate of Socrates; the question of Simon's historicity is not settled, cf. SellSS *passim*.

117 Read *taʿarrafa* (instead of *yuʿrafu*) *bihī*.

118 Arabic *Dīmuqrāṭīs* < *Δημόκριτος*, a 'pre-Socratic' Greek philosopher (d. ca. 370 BCE). Llavero Ruiz wrongly states "fue discípulo de Aristóteles, vivía a comienzos del 459 a.C. [!]", see ŶulGen 113 note 41.

119 Democritus hailed from Abdera, an ancient city on the Thracian coast.

120 This is a reference to the physio-philosophical concept known as 'atomism', with whose theoretical formulation Democritus is credited, alongside his teacher Leucippus. Unlike Leucippus, Democritus was a prolific writer, but his ideas have only survived in the form of more or less extensive fragments and quotations.

﴿٣٤﴾ The **third generation:** Greek sages who lived in the [Hellenistic] realm after the [ancient] Persians, and who were renowned in [the fields of] medicine and philosophy

Having mentioned the early sages who lived at the time of the [As]syrian and Persian empire[s],[121] before the Flood and thereafter, we must now turn to the third generation of sages, [those who lived] when hellenized states ruled over people—this period [covers] 242 years, beginning with Alexander and ending with the wise Cleopatra.[122] In Alexander's time, there were a large number of sages, among them[123] Andromachus,[124] Magnus of Emesa,[125] Diocles,[126] Paulus,[127] and others; they are less well known than the preceding ones but still deserve our notice, so that their turn is not forgotten. Among those who were famous in this era for [their contributions to] rational philosophy, stellar motions, and pioneering scientific discoveries are

---

121 My translation "(As)syrian and Persian empire(s)" is contextual: Ibn Juljul uses the phrase *al-dawla al-suryāniyya wa-l-kisrawāniyya* (lit. "the Syrian and Khosrowan [scil. Sasanian] empire[s]") which, looking at the opening chapters of his book, makes no chronological nor geographical sense as such.

122 The period described here by Ibn Juljul as beginning with (the death of) Alexander the Great and ending with (the death of) Cleopatra is what we call the 'Hellenistic' period (323–30 BCE, covering 293 [solar] years); Ibn Juljul's calculation of 242 (lunar) years seems to be based, despite his mention of Alexander, on the beginning of the reign of Ptolemy (see biography **12** below) through to the beginning of the reign of Cleopatra, covering 233 solar or 240 lunar years (284–51 BCE). Note that the name "Cleopatra" is represented here and in the following by ايلاو بيطره which should be emended to read قلاو بطره (*Qalāwbaṭrah* < *Κλεοπάτρα*), that is Cleopatra VII Philopator (d. 30 BCE).

123 The following short list of 'sages' shows that Ibn Juljul's immediately preceding remark, which places them "in Alexander's time" (*fī zaman al-Iskandar*), must be understood in an extremely wide sense, covering in effect the entire period from Alexander right down to Late Antiquity. As we shall see, this chapter on the 'third generation' is overall rather precarious in terms of chronology and biographical coherence; however, the associative dates given by Llavero Ruiz for Andromachus, Magnus of Emesa and Diocles are certainly wrong (ŶulGen 113 notes 43, 44 and 45).

124 Arabic *Andrumākhush* < *Ἀνδρόμαχος*, that is Andromachus the Elder, court physician to Nero (reg. 54–68 CE).

125 Arabic *Māghnush al-Ḥimṣī* (*Magnus Emesensis*), a physician who lived in the late 4th century CE and may be identical with Magnus of Nisibis who taught in Alexandria.

126 Arabic *Dhiyūqlish* < *Διοκλῆς*, that is Diocles of Carystus, also known as *Diocles Medicus* (d. ca. 295 BCE).

127 Arabic *Būlush* < *Παῦλος*, that is Paul of Aegina (fl. 7th century CE).

﴿٣٥﴾ 12
Ptolemy[128]

He ruled after Alexander.[129] He was desirous of knowledge, nay, crazy about it. He did a lot of research into the affairs of [ancient] kings and their biographies. [As] he was keen to discover the truth about the founding of Babylon and the story of Nimrod,[130] ﴿٣٦﴾ he inquired into this [matter] and, having located [the object of] his desire among the Israelites in Jerusalem, he sent to them Jerome the translator,[131] who rendered for him the *Torah* from Hebrew into Greek—there, he found the name of Nimrod and his story. Throughout his dominion he dispatched philosophers, so that they may measure for him the diameter of [his] land, and[132] its farthest inhabited or un[inhabited] regions. He observed the stars, and spoke about astronomy. On this [subject] he wrote his book known as *Almagest*; on the [subject of] climes he wrote his book known as *Geography*; and on stellar motions he wrote his *Canon*, which he based on the longitude of the clime he inhabited, namely the longitude of Alexandria, his city.[133]

He grasped the importance of medicine and philosophy, at whose development his contemporaries and their predecessors excelled. His teacher in [all] this was Aratus the astronomer,[134] who had no equal in terms of erudition. According to Orosius, [Ptolemy] ruled for 38 [solar] years.[135]

---

128 Arabic *Baṭalmiyūs* < *Πτολεμαῖος*, that is Ptolemy II Philadelphus, also known as Ptolemy the Great, pharaoh of Egypt (reg. 284–246 BCE).

129 Ptolemy II was the *second* Ptolemaic ruler, following his father, the Macedonian general Ptolemy I Soter.

130 Cf. note 20 above.

131 Cf. note 5 above. Ibn Juljul's assertion is chronologically impossible, as Jerome died in 420 CE (!).

132 Read *wa-jihātahā* (instead of *jihātahā*).

133 This 'bibliographical' passage represents a confusion between Ptolemy the pharaoh and Claudius Ptolemy, the famous Greco-Roman scientist who lived in Alexandria and died ca. 170 CE. *Claudius Ptolemy* is the author of the works cited here by Ibn Juljul: the "Almagest" (*Ἡ Μεγίστη* > *al-Majisṭī*); the "Geography" (*Γεωγραφικὴ* [*ὑφήγησις*] > *al-Jughrāfiya*); and the "Canon" or so-called 'Handy Tables' ([*Πρόχειροι*] *κανόνες* > *al-Qānūn*).

134 Arabic *Arāṭūs* < *Ἄρατος*, that is Aratus of Soloi (d. ca. 240 BCE), author of an extremely popular astronomical poem titled *Φαινόμενα*, dealing with constellations, celestial phenomena, and weather lore; he is also said to have been a physician, grammarian, and philosopher. Although his association with Ptolemy II is chronologically possible, Aratus is not known to have spent any time in Egypt, never mind as a 'teacher' (*muʿallim*) of the pharaoh. Llavero Ruiz (ŶulGen 114 note 52), after the editor of the Arabic text, considers to read *Aristarchus* (of Samos, d. ca. 230 BCE) instead of *Aratus*, but this would require a fairly radical emendation (ارسطرخس < اراطوس).

135 On Orosius and his *Histories* cf. note 4 above; the duration of Ptolemy's reign is correctly quoted by Ibn Juljul from the specified source, see OrKit 201 [154].

﴿٣٨﴾ 13
Cato[136]

the philosopher, master of numbers and measurement[s]. He lived during [the reign of] this dynasty, [namely] in the days of Ptolemy Dionysus.[137] His writing on arithmetic is known among the barbarians[138] as *Cato's Book for Cleopatra*,[139] the learned philosopher-queen;[140] he [also] dedicated to her [his] *Synoptic Canon*,[141] which is an unpretentious chart, easy to use [and] meeting the requirements.[142]

﴿٣٩﴾ 14
Euclid[143]

the master of geometry who, [coming] from the science of philosophy, proceeded on his own to study geometrical forms, in their basic as well as complex manifestations. [It happened that] one of the rulers of this Greek dynasty[144] came across two books in the libraries which were attributed to a man called Apollonius the carpenter,[145] who mentioned therein the structure of the five

---

136 Arabic *Qaṭūn* (through Latin?), a man of uncertain identity; cf. note 142 below.

137 Arabic *Baṭalmiyūs Diyūnīsūs* (thus, instead of دنونيسيوس) < *Πτολεμαῖος Διόνυσος*, that is Ptolemy XII Dionysus, also known as Ptolemy Auletes, pharaoh of Egypt (reg. 80–58 and 55–51 BCE) and father of Cleopatra VII Philopator.

138 That is, non-Arabic speakers, and more specifically speakers of Greek or Latin.

139 *Kitāb Qaṭūn ilā Qalāwbaṭrah* (thus, instead of ايلاويطره) < Greek/Latin title?

140 On Cleopatra cf. note 122 above.

141 *al-Qānūn al-mukhtaṣar* < Greek/Latin title?

142 The "Synoptic Canon" seems to have been some kind of ready reckoner. As regards the identity of *Cato*, we can only repeat the obvious and say that he must have been a Greek or, more likely, Roman mathematician of the 1st century BCE; the Arab bio-bibliographer al-Qifṭī (d. 646/1248) calls him *Fṭwn* "of the numbers" (*al-ʿadadī*), adding that the name of this "Greek sage" (*ḥakīm yūnānī*) is spelled by some with *Q* instead of *F* (undotted Arabic ڡ), see QifTaʾ 259. It is tempting, though chronologically impossible, to consider *Qṭwn* a misspelling of *Κόνων* (قنون instead of قطون), and thereby a reference to the Greek mathematician Conon of Samos, court astronomer to Ptolemy III Euergetes (reg. 246–222 BCE); equally tempting, though chronologically even more impossible, is to regard *Qṭwn* a misspelling of *Μέτων* (مطون instead of قطون), scil. Meton of Athens, a Greek astronomer, mathematician and geometer who lived in the 5th century BCE.

143 Arabic *Uqlīdis* < *Εὐκλείδης*, the famous Greek mathematician (fl. 300 BCE).

144 That is, the Ptolemaic dynasty. The ruler at whose Alexandrian court Euclid was active is Ptolemy I Soter, satrap and later pharaoh of Egypt (reg. 323–282 BCE).

145 Arabic *Abulūniyūs* < *Ἀπολλώνιος*, that is Apollonius of Perga, a Greek geometrician most

objects which may be enclosed in a sphere;[146] and [when] that ruler was looking for someone to help him solve [the problems posed by] these two books, he found no other than Euclid [who was the most knowledgeable geometrician of his time[147]]. So [Euclid] explained and interpreted for him the content of the two books, guiding him towards [an understanding of] their author's intention; then he presented the ruler with an introduction intended to teach [him] the structure of these solids. This is how the writing which is connected to [the name of] Euclid came into existence—in it, he begins by mentioning [the basics] that at the end combine to form [mathematical] proofs.[148] Thus it is related by Abū Yūsuf Yaʿqūb ibn Isḥāq al-Kindī in one of his epistles, from which I have been quoting literally.[149]

﴿٤١﴾ The **fourth generation:** Greek sages[150] who spoke during the Imperial Era, after the founding of Rome[151]

famous for his writing on conic sections titled *Κωνικά* (> *al-Makhrūṭāt*); his epithet 'the carpenter' (*al-najjār*) is a widespread (Arabic) interpolation, which is sometimes also extended to Euclid (e.g. QifTa' 62 and *passim*); he died in Alexandria around 190 BCE. Contrary to Ibn Juljul's subsequent account, it was Apollonius who elaborated on the earlier work of Euclid, and not the other way around.

146 This is a reference to the five regular polyhedra or so-called Platonic solids (cf. note 86 above)—the vertices of each solid, when projected into a sphere, all touch its circumference.

147 This is an addition to Ibn Juljul's original, obtained from two later sources and inserted by the editor of the Arabic text, for reasons not explained, see JulṬab 39 note 4.

148 This is no doubt an allusion to Euclid's chef-d'œuvre, the "Elements" (*Στοιχεῖα* > *al-Arkān* et al.)—to repeat: Apollonius' *Conics* are based on Euclid's *Elements*, not vice versa.

149 This is a reference to al-Kindī's (d. ca. 256/870) lost epistle (*risāla*) titled *Fī Aghrāḍ* (*kutub*) *Uqlīdis* "On the Objectives (of the books) of Euclid". There is no way to tell whether Ibn Juljul's version of this story is obtained directly from al-Kindī's original, or whether it is based on a secondary transmission; for two (more detailed) versions of the same story see NadFih 1/266,9–14 and QifTa' 63,7–22. Despite some narrative differences, all Arab authors maintain that Apollonius *preceded* Euclid.

150 This chapter does, in fact, deal exclusively with Galen.

151 Between the (legendary) founding of Rome and the end of the Imperial Era lies more than a millennium.

15
Galen[152]

He who is a native of the city of Pergamon.[153] This city belongs to the land of Asia[154] [and lies] east of Constantinople;[155] it is an island in the Sea of Constantinople.[156] Those [who live there] are Eastern Greco-Romans. From this corner [of the world], the race known among the Romans as 'Goths' broke forth, who [later] plundered al-Andalus and made it their home.[157]

Isidore[158] of Seville, the metropolitan [bishop], mentions that the city of Pergamon was the site of a royal prison, where [the kings] used to detain those with whom they were angry.[159] This [our] Galen lived during the reign

152 Arabic *Jālīnūs* < *Γαληνός*, the famous Greek physician (d. 216 CE).

153 Arabic *Birghamush* < *Πέργαμον/ς*, an ancient Greek city in Mysia.

154 That is, Asia *Minor*.

155 Arabic (*madīnat*) *Qusṭanṭīniyya* < *Κωνσταντινούπολις*. Strictly speaking, Pergamon lies *west* of Constantinople.

156 Pergamon is not an 'island' (*jazīra*); the 'Sea of Constantinople' (*baḥr Qusṭanṭīniyya*) is the Sea of Marmara.

157 *al-Qūṭ* is a generic name for "Goths"; it is possible, though perhaps unlikely, that Ibn Juljul's short statement dimly reflects a notional distinction between Ostrogoths and Visigoths, the latter becoming the founders of the Visigothic Kingdom of Toledo (6th to early 8th centuries CE). In Ibn Juljul's days, al-Andalus denoted the entire Muslim-ruled area of the Iberian Peninsula.

158 Read *Ishīdur* (instead of *Bshyr*).

159 Isidore of Seville (Arabic *Ishīdur* [et al.] *al-Ishbīlī*, d. 636 CE) was a Spanish cleric and polymath who authored, among various other writings, a sweeping, highly influential encyclopedia titled *Origines* or, as it is distinguished by a predilection for etymological and lexicological explanations, *Etymologiae*—for the Latin *editio princeps* see IsEty, for an English translation see EtyIs. Ibn Juljul's above 'quotation' cannot be traced to Isidore's chef-d'œuvre, which surely would have constituted his most likely source; there is, moreover, no record of an Arabic translation of this work. However, it is hardly conceivable that Ibn Juljul simply invented this reference and/or fabricated the information that goes along with it—Fu'ād Sayyid, the editor of the *Ṭabaqāt*, maintains that the passage in question is indeed a quotation from a (lost) Arabic translation of Isidore's *Origins* (JulṬab [avant-propos] 9); Manfred Ullmann is much more sceptical and considers Sayyid's proposal to be baseless (UllMed 230 note 2); and Juan Vernet, having pointed out the possibility of oral transmissions, adds that selected segments of the work may well have existed in Arabic translation (VerMA 452 with note 64). In fact, as Vernet also already indicated (loc.cit.), we do possess a number of examples from Arabic geographical literature that clearly imply the existence of at least partial translations of Isidore's *Origins*—the Arab Andalusian historian and geographer Abū 'Ubayd al-Bakrī (d. 487/1094), in his *Kitāb al-Masālik wa-l-mamālik* "Book of Highways and Kingdoms", offers several entries that depend on Isidore's work; the editor of these passages, Jean-Charles Ducène, concludes his study with the following remarks: "Il est undéniable que ces passages d'al-Bakrī provi-

of Nero[160] Caesar, who was the sixth of the Caesars that ruled Rome.[161] [Galen] widely roamed [foreign] lands and, having moved to Rome twice, he [finally] settled down there. He accompanied its emperor on military campaigns, looking after the wounded. He excelled at medicine, philosophy and all physical sciences [already] at the age of seventeen, and he became an authority [in these fields] when he was twenty-four. He updated the knowledge of Hippocrates and wrote commentaries on those of his books which he had studied but which were difficult to understand for his contemporaries.[162] He held public[163] meetings in the city of Rome, where he gave lectures ﴾٤٢﴿ [in which] he proved and displayed his well-known, extraordinary grasp of anatomy. He [produced] a large number of writings on [various] branches of science. His father was a building surveyor, and nobody in his time knew more about surveying than he did. The religion of Christianity had [already] emerged in [Galen's] days.

It was said to him: "In Jerusalem, at the end of Caesar Octavian's reign,[164] a man had[165] appeared who cured the blind and the leper, and who brought the dead back to life". [Galen] replied: "In order to accomplish this, he must have had almost divine power"; and then he asked: "Are any of his followers still around?" When the answer was "Yes", he left Rome, aiming for Jerusalem.

---

ennent des *Étymologies* d'Isidore de Séville [...] Pour en revenir au texte d'Isidore, on peut remarquer un flottement entre le texte latin et le texte arabe qui parfois s'éloigne du texte à traduire ou l'abrège [...] Effectivement, si aucune traduction arabe de cet ouvrage n'a encore été retrouvée, il faut cependant noter l'existence de plusieurs manuscrits latins wisigothiques comportant de nombreuses gloses en arabe" (DucIs 391ff.). It is therefore absolutely possible that Ibn Juljul had access to Arabic segments of Isidore's work, and that these segments contained secondary amplifications along the lines evidenced above. Finally, the question of whether or not there was a 'royal prison' (*sijn al-mulūk*) in Pergamon, is impossible to answer—IAU 3.1/208 note 98, this claim is considered "apocryphal" by the editors.

160 Read *Nīrū* (instead of *Qyra*, undotted Arabic ٮٮرو / ڡٮره); this is a chronological blunder, as Nero reigned from 54–68 CE, decades before the birth of Galen. Another possible emendation is to read *Tibirah* "Tiberius" (undotted Arabic ٮٮره), but this would take us even further back in time, clashing moreover with the immediately following specification. Cf. also ŶulGen 115 note 59.

161 Nero was the *fifth* emperor of the Julio-Claudian dynasty, but Ibn Juljul (or his source) may have counted from Gaius Julius Caesar.

162 For a list of Galenic commentaries on Hippocratic writings see UllMed 61f. and GaS 3/123f.

163 Read *ʿāmma* (instead of *ʿāmmiyya*).

164 That is Caesar Augustus, also known as Octavian (Arabic *Uktabiyān*), the first Roman emperor of the Julio-Claudian dynasty (reg. 27 BCE–14 CE).

165 The insertion of the perfect particle *qad* is an appropriate editorial intervention.

He got as far as Sicily, which in those days was called Sicania,[166] but there he died, and there is his grave. He lived 88 years.[167]

He is the key to medicine—he greatly developed and thoroughly interpreted it, after [his] predecessors. His is a collection of sixteen interconnected [writings][168] which the student of medicine is obliged to memorize and to utilize, if he seeks to learn this science without [the burden of clinical] proof[s]. The first of them is his book [titled] *On the Schools of Medicine*, then his book *On the Elements*, then his book *On the Mixture*, then his book *On Simple Drugs*, then his book *On Compound Drugs*, then his book *On Causes and Symptoms*, then his book *On Afflicted Organs*, then his book *On the Method*[169] *of Healing*, then his book *On the Natural Powers*, then his epistle *To Glaucon*, then his book *On the Converging Opinions of Hippocrates and Plato*, then his book *On the Crisis*, then his book *On the Days of the Crisis*, then his book *On Fevers*, then his book *On the Kinds of Fevers*,[170] then his book *To Teuthras*[171] *on the Pulse*.[172]

---

166 Sicania (Arabic *Ṣikāniyah*), so called after its ancient inhabitants, the *Σικανοί*.

167 Galen was born in 129 CE, and the current consensus is that he died in 216 CE, aged *87*.

168 This is a reference to the so-called *Summaria Alexandrinorum*—for more details see note 172 below.

169 Read *ḥīla* (instead of *ḥlya*, a printing error).

170 This writing is, in fact, identical with the preceding one (i.e. *Aṣnāf al-ḥummayāt* and *al-Ḥummayāt* are variant titles of the same Galenic text, cf. UllMed 42 no. 24 and 66f.); perhaps Ibn Juljul's reading *aṣnāf* "kinds" is a mistake for *adwār* "periods", and thereby a reference to Galen's *Πρὸς τοὺς περὶ τύπων γράψαντας ἢ περὶ περιόδων* (Arabic *Fī Adwār al-ḥummayāt wa-tarākībihā* [FiCG 45f. no. 52]).

171 Arabic *Ṭūtharā* (elsewhere *Ṭūtharan*) < *Τεύθρας*, a fellow-student and old friend of Galen.

172 This 'collection' (here: *dīwān* [!]) of sixteen Galenic writings is otherwise known in Arabic as *Jawāmiʿ al-Iskandarāniyyīn*, Latin *Summaria Alexandrinorum*, a didactically arranged canon that was put together by a number of Alexandrian physicians, probably in the 5th or 6th century CE; the Greek original of the *Summaria* is lost, and mentioned nowhere in subsequent Greek works; the literary genesis and transmissional history of this compilation is extremely complicated, and Arab authors give different accounts regarding the precise content and sequential organization of the *Summaria*—for a tabular synopsis, illustrating the complexity of the problem, see UllMed 343; for a general overview cf. op.cit. 65ff. and GaS 3/140–150. It is worth noting that further down, when he discusses the **fifth generation**, Ibn Juljul offers us his own brief version of the story, and there more aptly refers to the *Summaria* by the Arabic terms *jumal wa-jawāmiʿ*. Returning, then, to Ibn Juljul's titular sequence of the *Summaria*, Arabic–Greek equations are as follows: *Fī Firaq al-ṭibb* < *Περὶ αἱρέσεων τοῖς εἰσαγομένοις*, *Fī l-Usṭuqussāt* < *Περὶ τῶν καθ' Ἱπποκράτην στοιχείων*, *Fī l-Mizāj* < *Περὶ κράσεων*, *Fī l-Adwiya al-mufrada* < *Περὶ κράσεως καὶ δυνάμεως τῶν ἁπλῶν φαρμάκων*, *Fī l-Adwiya al-murakkaba* < *Περὶ συνθέσεως φαρμάκων*, *Fī l-ʿIlal wa-l-aʿrāḍ* < *Περὶ διαφορᾶς νοσημάτων* + *Περὶ τῶν ἐν τοῖς νοσήμασιν*

On him who wants to learn medicine together with [clinical] proof[s], another condition is imposed [by Galen], and explained most clearly in his book [titled] *On the Order of Reading that which he [Wrote]*.[173]

This [our] Galen knew how to furnish a [clinical] proof; he [also] spoke well in public. His is a book in which he contradicts the poets,[174] and another [titled] *On Faulty Speech of Common People*.[175] Nobody surpassed his knowledge of anatomy—on this [subject] he composed [a book in] seventeen parts [titled] *On the Dissection of Dead Beings*, as well as a book [titled] *On the Dissection of Living Beings*.[176] He wrote commentaries on all writings of Hippocrates and interpreted them.[177] He [also] composed a book [titled] *On Gymnastics with the Small Ball*.[178]

In his time, there was a group of people who related to the science of Aristotle. They ran under the name 'companions ﴿٤٣﴾ of the shaded place'; these are the Stoics.[179] Against them, [Galen] composed a book [titled] *On Cohes-*

αἰτιῶν + *Περὶ τῶν συμπτωμάτων διαφορᾶς* + *Περὶ αἰτιῶν συμπτωμάτων*, *Fī l-Aʿḍāʾ al-ālima* < *Περὶ τῶν πεπονθότων τόπων*, *Fī Ḥīlat al-burʾ* < *Θεραπευτικὴ μέθοδος*, *Fī l-Quwā l-ṭabīʿiyya* < *Περὶ φυσικῶν δυνάμεων*, *Ilā Ighlawqun* < *Πρὸς Γλαύκωνα θεραπευτικά*, *Fī ʾttifāq ārāʾ Buqrāṭ wa-Aflāṭun* < *Περὶ τῶν Ἱπποκράτους καὶ Πλάτωνος δογμάτων*, *Fī l-Buḥrān* < *Περὶ κρίσεων*, *Fī Ayyām al-buḥrān* < *Περὶ κρισίμων ἡμερῶν*, *Fī l-Ḥummayāt* / *Fī Aṣnāf al-ḥummayāt* (cf. note 170 above) < *Περὶ διαφορᾶς πυρετῶν*, *Fī l-Nabḍ ilā Ṭūtharā* < *Περὶ τῶν σφυγμῶν τοῖς εἰσαγομένοις*. All these works had become available in Arabic translations by the middle of the 3rd/9th century, see (in the sequence given above) FiCG 10ff. no. 4, 15f. no. 8, 16 no. 9, 63 no. 78, 64f. nos 80 and 82, 41ff. nos 42, 43, 44 and 45, 50f. no. 60, 56ff. no. 69, 17 no. 10, 58f. no. 70, 33ff. no. 33, 55 no. 67, 55f. no. 68, 44 no. 48 (and perhaps 45f. no. 52), 51f. no. 61.

173 *Fī Marātib mā yuqraʾu lahū*, properly known as *Fī Marātib qirāʾat kutubihī* "On the Order of Reading his Books" < *Περὶ τῆς τάξεως τῶν ἰδίων βιβλίων*, see FiCG 82 no. 115.

174 *kitāb nāqaḍa fīhi l-shuʿarāʾ* (?).

175 *Fī Laḥn al-ʿāmma* < *Πρὸς τοὺς ἐπιτιμῶντας τοῖς σολοικίζουσι τῇ φωνῇ*, see BergGÜ 42 no. 129; the work is only known from Galen's autobibliography, see FiCG 91 no. 136.

176 *Fī Tashrīḥ al-mawtā* < *Περὶ τῆς ἐπὶ τῶν τεθνεώτων ἀνατομῆς* and, respectively, *Fī Tashrīḥ al-aḥyāʾ* < *Περὶ τῆς ἐπὶ τῶν ζώντων ἀνατομῆς*, see FiCG 97 nos 169 and 171. It is not clear where Ibn Juljul's specification 'seventeen parts' (*sabʿ ʿashara maqāla*) comes from—according to Ḥunayn ibn Isḥāq, the work in question consisted of just one part. Perhaps Ibn Juljul confused it with Galen's main anatomical work, the *ʿIlāj al-tashrīḥ* or *al-Tashrīḥ al-kabīr* < *Ἀνατομικαὶ ἐγχειρήσεις*, which at least consisted of fifteen parts, see BergGÜ 15f. no. 21 with FiCG 18f. no. 11; taken together, the individual parts of these three works add up to eighteen (1, 2, 15).

177 Cf. note 162 above.

178 *Fī l-Kura al-ṣaghīra wa-l-riyāḍa bi-hā* < *Περὶ τοῦ διὰ μικρᾶς σφαίρας γυμνασίου*, see FiCG 36 no. 35.

179 The 'shaded place' (*miẓalla*) is a reference to the colonnades in the Agora of Athens,

ive Causes,[180] because it was they who claimed that the pneuma is a cohesive cause.[181] Regarding phlebotomy, [Galen] disagreed with Erasistratus,[182] just as he refuted many of [his] predecessors; he [also] disagreed with the Sophists. On logic, he composed a book [titled] *The Proof*,[183] and against medical tricksters he composed a book [too].[184]

In his book [titled] *On Diseases that are Difficult to Cure*,[185] [Galen] says that as he was walking through the city of Rome, he came across a man who, surrounded by a group of fools, shouted: 'I am a native of Aleppo! I have met Galen and he has taught me everything he knows, all of it! Here is a useful remedy against tooth-worms!' The lowlife had already prepared a hazelnut[-sized lump] made from pitch and tar, which he now placed over embers. With this, he fumigated the mouth of a bystander who had declared to have wormy teeth. The man could not help closing his eyes, and when he had done so, [the charlatan] inserted into his mouth some worms which he kept ready in boxes. Then he extracted them from the mouth of the dental patient. No sooner had he accomplished this [feat], than the fools showered him with their [coins]. Finally, he outdid himself by cutting into veins away from joints. "When I saw this" [Galen continues] "I revealed myself to the crowd, saying: 'I am Galen! And that one is a shameless, lying idiot!' Then I warned them off him, and reported him to the authorities". In this way, [Galen] thwarted [the charlatan], and for that reason he composed a book on tricksters.[186]

---

where the Stoic philosophers used to gather; the Arabic word for 'Stoics' (*riwāqiyyūn* "those of the portico") is derived from *riwāq*, itself a loan-translation of *στοά* "roofed colonnade".

180 *Fī l-Asbāb al-māsika* < *Περὶ τῶν συνεκτικῶν αἰτιῶν*, see FiCG 100 f. no. 187.

181 For a discussion of this problem see CouCC 259 ff. and *passim*.

182 This is almost certainly a reference to Galen's polemical work *Περὶ φλεβοτομίας πρὸς Ἐρασίστρατον* and, by extension, *Περὶ φλεβοτομίας πρὸς Ἐρασιστρατείους τοὺς ἐν Ῥώμῃ*, see FiCG 59 f. nos 71 and 72 with GaS 3/115 no. 57. Erasistratus was a Greek anatomist and physiologist who died around 250 BCE. Ibn Juljul's *ʾsqlybyāds* (scil. Asclepiades) is to be emended accordingly.

183 *al-Burhān* < *Περὶ ἀποδείξεων*, see FiCG 105 f. no. 209.

184 This is probably a reference to *Περὶ μεθοδικῆς αἱρέσεως*, in which Galen attacked the doctrines of the Methodics (here: *aṣḥāb al-ḥiyal*) for their therapeutic simplifications; the work is only known from Galen's autobibliography, see FiCG 117 no. 271.

185 *Fī l-Amrāḍ al-ʿasīrat al-burʾ* < **Περὶ δυσιάτων νοσημάτων**, see FiCG 152 no. 439 (lost in Greek). The earliest *reference* to this work in Arabic literature is found in Qusṭā ibn Lūqā's (d. 300/912) Galen-bibliography, see MeySch 17 no. 29; the following *story*, however, was first recorded by Ibn Juljul.

186 For a parallel version of this story, based (implicitly) on Ibn Juljul's account, see IAU 3.1/217; for Galen's writing on 'tricksters' (*aṣḥāb al-ḥiyal*) cf. note 184 above.

In the book *Qāṭājānis*,[187] [Galen] mentions that he operated in[188] a temple in the city of Rome, having taken over from an older master who had been [working] there—this [temple] was in effect a hospital where the wounded were treated. All those on whom he—ahead of others—operated, triumphed [over their injuries].[189] This is how [Galen's] superiority became obvious, and his knowledge apparent. He was never content to learn things only by rote, without direct practice.

He travelled to Cyprus to see chalcanthite[190] in its mine, and he also travelled to the island of Chios[191] to see the discovery site of sealing bole—all these [products] he handled for himself and verified through inspection.

According to his own account, none of his contemporaries showed a greater devotion to the study of books than he did—every day, he applied himself to learning a piece of wisdom; [then], in the evening, he betook himself to [his] teachers, submitting to them his [knowledge] for examination.[192] Before long, his companions and fellows nicknamed him 'word-smith' and ﴾٤٤﴿ 'wonder-talker'. As he mentions at the beginning of [his] book *The Method*[193] *of Healing*, he did not accept a thing from the kings, nor trust them, nor seek their company.[194] He was extremely critical of all [other] writers, and not a single one of [his literary] predecessors escaped unscathed.

This, then, is the portrait of Galen, and [such was] the calibre of the man and his knowledge. Were it not for him, medicine would have vanished, it would have become extinct and fallen into oblivion all over the world. Yet he kept

---

187 This is a reference to *Περὶ συνθέσεως φαρμάκων τῶν κατὰ γένη*, a Galenic work on pharmacology arranged according to drug categories (rather than afflicted organs), see FiCG 64f. no. 82; the full Arabic title is *Tarkīb al-adwiya ʿalā l-jumal wa-l-ajnās*, but it was also known as *Qāṭājānis*, which is a transliteration of *κατὰ γένη*.

188 The insertion of the preposition *fī* is an appropriate editorial intervention.

189 This short passage is a heavily warped, radically abridged representation of GOO 13/599f. (... *κατὰ γένη*), dealing primarily with the treatment of wounded *gladiators*. Is Ibn Juljul's 'temple' (*haykal*) a reference to the Colosseum?

190 Arabic *al-khalqaṭārā/ī* < *τὸ χάλκανθον* or, possibly, < *ἡ χαλκῖτις* "calcite".

191 Perhaps read *Limnūs* "Lemnos" instead of *Kiyūsh* "Chios" (undotted Arabic لمنوس / كىوس).

192 This is a selective paraphrase of a longer passage in Galen's *Miḥnat al-ṭabīb* "The Examination of the Physician" (lost in Greek, see FiCG 110f. no. 232), in which he describes his own work ethics and clinical approach, not sparing his contemporaries from scorn, see IskGal 100–105 (Arabic text and English translation).

193 Read *ḥīla* (instead of *ḥlya*, a printing error).

194 I have not been able to trace this 'quotation' to Ibn Juljul's specified source, scil. *Ḥīlat al-burʾ* < *Θεραπευτικὴ μέθοδος* (FiCG 56ff. no. 69).

it alive, elucidated its mysteries, and made its difficulties easy [to understand]. There were [other] philosophers in his time, but their memory has been effaced by his, and even their names are now forgotten.

﴿٥١﴾ The **fifth generation:** Alexandrian sages

After the era of Christ—peace be upon him—had come, when his message had spread throughout the lands of the Romans and when all of them had converted to Christianity, a group of experienced philosophers emerged in Alexandria, who systematically inspected their stock of old books. Then they abridged the entirety of Galen's writings, without changing their basic contents, and turned them into epitomes and summaries, so that they may be easier to memorize and to understand.[195] Ḥunayn the translator[196] had these writings at his disposal, in their original as well as in their summarized forms,[197] and so they are still found to this day. The head of the Alexandrians was Anqīlāwus of Alexandria.[198] It was he who compiled from the words of the famous Galen a tome in thirteen treatises.[199] He [also] wrote a book [titled] *On the Secrets of Movements*, dedicated to [the benefit of] those who engage in sexual intercourse whilst suffering from one or another chronic illness; in this [book] he mentions what arouses [a desire] for [sex], and what wards off its [potential]

195 On the so-called *Summaria Alexandrinorum* cf. note 172 above. Earlier on, in his biography of Galen (15), Ibn Juljul speaks of (and records) sixteen *specific* writings, and does not imply *abridgements* of any kind.

196 That is, Ḥunayn ibn Isḥāq al-ʿIbādī (d. 260/873 or 264/877), the famous Nestorian Arab physician and translator from Greek and Syriac, on whom see e.g. StrḤu *passim*.

197 In his account of translated Galenic writings, Ḥunayn frequently refers to the Alexandrian redaction, too, see the passages registered in BergGÜ 44 s.n. *Alexandrien*; on one occasion, he moreover refers to their identity and redactorial sequence, see op.cit. 15,4–15.

198 The name Anqīlāwus is difficult to etymologize, never mind substantiate historically. It may well be, as has already been suggested (IAU 3.1/276 note 7), a corruption of Nicolaus (*Niqūlāwus* < *Νικόλαος*, undotted Arabic يعولاوس / ابعـلاوس), but that does not take us much further. Irvine and Temkin cautiously opt for an identification of Anqīlāwus with Ἀγγελεύας "in the Greek text of Stephanos's [of Athens, fl. ca. 600 CE] *Commentary on Galen's Therapeutics to Glaucon*" (ITAk 14–18 [esp. p. 15]), but there is no certainty here either.

199 This statement probably means that Anqīlāwus redacted thirteen of the sixteen writings that combine to form the *Summaria Alexandrinorum*—an interpretation which is upheld also by Fuat Sezgin, see GaS 3/160.

damage[200]—with God's permission. From among those [scholars], his name is [the most] widely known, but they numbered many.[201]

﴿٥٣﴾ The **sixth generation**: those who were not of Greco-Roman, nor Syrian, nor Persian descent[202]

After God had revealed Islam and the message of our prophet Muḥammad—may He bless him and grant him salvation—had spread far and wide, all other [spiritual] callings were silenced by it; this was during the reign of the emperor Heraclius,[203] who had set up camp in Syria, in [the city of] Antioch.[204] Then God raised the word of strong faith and the banner of true guidance: supreme dynastic power, superior lordship and profound higher wisdom fell to the Arabs, and all [once] victorious dynasties as well as all existing religious communities were gradually subdued. For [Muḥammad], God chose Yathrib[205] as a residence, the Hejaz as a safe region, and the 'helpers'[206] as companions.

Among the sages [and] physicians of illustrious renown and unconcealed fame who lived in the days of the Messenger of God[207]—may He bless him and grant him salvation—are

200 The work *Fī Asrār al-ḥarakāt* "On the Secrets of Movements" (also recorded QifTa' 71,11 f.) is probably a pseudepigraph; the Arabic version of this text is lost, and so is its Greek *Vorlage*, if there ever was one.

201 According to most Arabic sources, there were *seven* redactors of the *Summaria Alexandrinorum*: Anqīlāwus, Stephanus, Gessius, Theodosius, Archelaus, Palladius and John Philoponus, see the discussion in GaS 3/140–146 and IAU 3.1/276 with notes 4–8; in a more general sense, Ibn Juljul's remark that "they numbered many" (*'adaduhum kathīr*) may of course also include 'generations' of Alexandrian scholars who were not directly, or not at all, involved in the redaction of the *Summaria*.

202 Note, however, that the fourth and last scholar of this 'generation', Māsarjawayh, is described by Ibn Juljul himself as a Syrian Jew (*yahūdī l-madhhab suryānī*), see biography 19 below.

203 Arabic *Hiraql* < *Ἡράκλειος*, that is the Byzantine emperor Flavius Heraclius (reg. 610–641 CE).

204 At one point during the early Arab-Byzantine wars, Heraclius was briefly in Antioch, see KaeByz 79; the city was eventually captured by Muslim armies in 637 CE, in the so-called Battle of the Iron Bridge.

205 Yathrib was the pre-Islamic name of the Arabian city of Medina.

206 *al-Anṣār* "The Helpers" were the local inhabitants of Yathrib-Medina who supported Muḥammad and his followers after their 'migration' (*hijra*) from Mecca in 622 CE, which event marks the beginning of the Islamic era.

207 This is, as we shall see and as Ibn Juljul himself later corroborates, chronologically true only for the first two sages of the present 'generation'.

﴿٥٤﴾ 16
al-Ḥārith

ibn Kalada al-Thaqafī.[208] He learned medicine in the territory of Persia and in Yemen, where he practised it [for a while]; he knew about drug[s]; he used to play the lute, which is something he also learned in Persia and in Yemen. He was alive in the days of the Messenger of God—may He bless him and grant him salvation; [he continued to live through] the days of Abū Bakr, ʿUmar, ʿUthmān, ʿAlī ibn Abī Ṭālib,[209] and Muʿāwiya[210]—may God be pleased with them.[211] [When] Muʿāwiya said to him: "What is medicine, O Ḥārith?", he replied: "Eating but once a day, O Commander of the Faithful", which is to say 'going hungry'.[212]

In the days of the Messenger of God—may He bless him and grant him salvation—there were physicians from the [Arab] tribe of Anmār. [It happened that the prophet]—may God bless him and grant him salvation—came to see one of his companions, who was wounded, and said to the two [attendant] physicians: "Which of you is more skilled in medicine?" [When] one of them replied: "I am, O Messenger of God!", he said: "In that case, you take over!" [And when] somebody asked him: "O Messenger of God! Is there a supreme healer?", he said: "Yes—it is He who sends down the remedy together with the illness". Then [the prophet]—may God bless him and grant him salvation—left, having given his approval.[213]

---

208 al-Ḥārith ibn Kalada al-Thaqafī, the "physician of the Arabs" (IAU 3.1/297,-1), was a contemporary of the prophet Muḥammad. al-Ḥārith died, according to some sources, in the decade between 13/634 and 23/644; according to others, he lived until at least the year 41/661. The latter estimate is also implied by Ibn Juljul's account. For more information about al-Ḥārith see UllMed 19 f., GaS 3/203 f. and InkḤā *passim*.

209 *ʿAlī ibn Abī Ṭālib* is a logical addition on the part of the editor of the Arabic text, who refers to the parallel passage IAU 3.1/296. Abū Bakr (al-Ṣiddīq), ʿUmar (ibn al-Khaṭṭāb), ʿUthmān (ibn ʿAffān) and ʿAlī ibn Abī Ṭālib are the names of the first four caliphs that succeeded the prophet Muḥammad; their combined reign covers the years 11/632–41/661.

210 Muʿāwiya ibn Abī Sufyān, also referred to as Muʿāwiya I, was the first caliph of the Umayyad dynasty; he reigned from 41/661 to 60/680.

211 This eulogy is a (probably justified) editorial addition.

212 The earliest version of this anecdote in Arabic literature seems to be found in ʿAlī ibn Sahl al-Ṭabarī's (d. between 246/860 and 256/870) "Book of the Pearl" (*Kitāb al-Luʾluʾa*), where the featured caliph is ʿUmar (instead of Muʿāwiya), see ṬabBP 42 f. § 4 (with note 9 for further sources and explanations). The 'definition' of medicine given by al-Ḥārith obviously boils down to the idea of dietary restraint.

213 A more coherent version of this anecdote is recorded by the orthodox theologian Ibn Qayyim al-Jawziyya (d. 751/1350) in his "Prophetic Medicine" (*al-Ṭibb al-nabawī*), on the authority of the 8th century CE traditionist Mālik ibn Anas, see IQNab 105. There is no tan-

When [the caliph] ʿUmar[214]—may God be pleased with him—lay wounded and was seen by a physician, [the latter] said: "Let him drink milk! If it comes out of his wound, he is bound to die". As the milk did come out of the wound, suggesting that [ʿUmar's] guts were injured, [the physician] said to him: "Arrange your affairs, for it will not take long before you join the buried". This [story] is transmitted on the authority of al-Ḥārith ibn Kalada.[215]

It is related on the authority of Saʿd ibn Abī Waqqāṣ,[216] who said: "When I was suffering from an illness, the Messenger of God—may He bless him and grant him salvation—visited me and said: 'Fetch al-Ḥārith ibn Kalada, for he knows about medicine!'"[217] Then the Messenger of God—may He bless him and grant him salvation—ordered to fetch [other] physicians and to ask their opinion about [the case] on hand.[218]

﴾٥٧﴿ 17
Ibn Abī Rimtha[219]

Skilled in the art of the hand,[220] he was a physician during the era of the Messenger of God—may He bless him and grant him salvation.

gible connection between the present anecdote and al-Ḥārith ibn Kalada, who belonged to the Arab tribe of Thaqīf. The phrase *anzala l-dawāʾ man anzala l-dāʾ* "He who sends down the remedy together with the illness" took on an independent existence in variously modified forms, along the lines of *mā anzala llāh^{u} dāʾ^{an} illā anzala lah^{u} dawāʾ^{an}* "God sends down no illness without sending down a remedy for it", cf. JulṬab 55 note 11 and ŶulGen 116 note 68.

214 Cf. note 209 above.

215 The editor of the Arabic text considers this anecdote to be an 'import' (*īrād*) of Ibn Juljul, see JulṬab 56 note 16.

216 Saʿd ibn Abī Waqqāṣ (d. ca. 50/670), a long-standing companion of the prophet Muḥammad and later commander of the Arab armies during the conquest of Iraq, see HawSW *passim*.

217 For the full version of this short anecdote, which ends with Saʿd's recovery, see IAU 3.1/298.

218 This final sentence is twisting in the wind.

219 Ibn Abī Rimtha was a physician from the Arab tribe of Tamīm and a contemporary of the prophet Muḥammad; he outlived the latter but the date of his death is not known, see UllMed 20 and GaS 3/204. His father, ʿUmāra ibn Yathrib (*Abū Rimtha*), was a prominent transmitter of prophetic traditions, see e.g. IḤMus 6/504–518 nos 7104–7118 and *passim*; Sezgin (GaS loc.cit.) confuses the two. Note that all later medical biographers depend on Ibn Juljul's above account.

220 That is to say surgery.

Nuʿaym relates on the authority of Ibn ʿUyayna[221] on the authority of Ibn Abjar[222] on the authority of Iyād ibn Laqīṭ[223] on the authority of Ibn Abī Rimtha,[224] who said:[225] "I came to the prophet—may God bless him and grant him salvation. [When] I noticed the seal[226] between his shoulder blades ﴿٥٨﴾ and said: 'I am a physician, let me treat this for you', he replied: 'You may well be skillful, but the physician is God'".[227] The Messenger of God—may He bless him and grant him salvation—understood that [Ibn Abī Rimtha] was manually skilled, yet limited in terms of [medical] knowledge—the proof lies in his words "but the physician is God".

Nuʿaym[228] relates that [when] Ubayy ibn Kaʿb[229] was suffering, the Messenger of God—may He bless him and grant him salvation—dispatched a physician to treat him.[230]

221 The text erroneously reads Ibn *Abī* ʿUyayna.

222 The text erroneously reads Ibn *Abḥar*.

223 The text erroneously reads *Ziyād ʿan* Laqīṭ.

224 Strictly speaking, the primary transmitter is *Abū Rimtha*, but his son eyewitnessed the scene and features, in fact, as its protagonist, cf. note 227 below.

225 The chain of transmitters is: Nuʿaym ibn Ḥammād al-Khuzāʿī (d. 228/843) ← Sufyān ibn ʿUyayna al-Hilālī (d. 198/814) ← ʿAbd al-Malik ibn Abjar al-Kinānī (see biography 18 below) ← Iyād ibn Laqīṭ al-Sadūsī ← Abū Rimtha / Ibn Abī Rimtha; on the dates of death of Nuʿaym and Sufyān see ʿAsTT 4/235b,-11f. and, respectively, 2/61a,-6f. This chain, introducing a different version of the following anecdote, is confirmed by the traditionist Aḥmad ibn Ḥanbal (d. 241/855), see IḤMus 13/389f. no. 17422; cf. also note 227 below.

226 That is the 'Seal (*khātim*) of Prophethood', here mistaken for a mole or growth. Applied as an epithet to Muḥammad, *khātim* signifies the "*Last* (of the Prophets)".

227 An older version of this anecdote (and presumably Ibn Juljul's source) reads as follows: [... on the authority of Abū Rimtha, who said] "I came to the Messenger of God—may He bless him and grant him salvation—together with my son [read *ibnī* instead of *abī*]; he noticed that thing on [the prophet's] back, and said: 'O Messenger of God! Shall I not treat this for you? I am a physician'. [The prophet] replied: 'You may well be skillful, but it is God who is the physician'. [Then] he said [to me]: 'Whom have you brought along with you there?', and I replied: 'My son (*ibnī*)'", see IḤMus 13/389f. no. 17422.

228 Cf. note 225 above.

229 Ubayy ibn Kaʿb al-Anṣārī (d. between 19/640 and 35/656), secretary to the prophet Muḥammad in Medina and early collector of the *Koran*, see RiUK *passim*.

230 One must assume that this physician was Ibn Abī Rimtha.

﴿٥٩﴾ 18
Ibn Abjar[231]

He was a knowledgeable, highly skilled physician who lived in the days of the Marwānids.[232] It is related that ʿUmar ibn ʿAbd al-ʿAzīz[233] used to send him his water.[234]

﴿٦١﴾ 19
Māsarjawayh[235]

He was a Syrian Jew. Under the Marwānid dynasty,[236] he completed an Arabic translation of the book of Ahrun ibn Aʿyan the presbyter.[237] [Later] ʿUmar ibn ʿAbd al-ʿAzīz[238] found [a copy of] it in [one of] the libraries, ordered it to be removed, and put it on his prayer mat; then he asked God for guidance as to whether he should make it available to the Muslims, so that they may benefit from it; after having reflected on this [matter] for forty[239] mornings, he did make it available to people, and [ensured] its distribution among them.

---

231 ʿAbd al-Malik ibn Abjar (not *Abḥar*, as the text erroneously reads) was a physician from the Arab tribe of Kinān, who died towards the end of the second decade of the 2nd/8th century, see UllMed 21 and GaS 3/205 f.

232 The Marwānids (*Banū Marwān*) are a branch of the Umayyad dynasty; their reign began with the accession of *Marwān* I ibn al-Ḥakam in 64/684 and lasted (in the Islamic East) until the ʿAbbāsid Revolution in 132/750. Ibn Juljul also refers to them as "the Marwānid dynasty" (*al-dawla al-Marwāniyya*), see the beginning of biography 19 below.

233 ʿUmar ibn ʿAbd al-ʿAzīz, also referred to as ʿUmar II, was the eighth caliph of the Umayyad dynasty; he reigned from 99/717 to 101/720.

234 That is, his urine.

235 Māsarjawayh (Persian Māsargōye), also known in Arabic as Māsarjīs, was a physician who seems to have been active in Basra during the decades between 680 and 720 CE, though even this rough estimate is not entirely uncontroversial, see UllMed 23 f., GaS 3/206 f. and DietMā *passim*.

236 Cf. note 232 above. It is possible, albeit less likely, that the phrase *al-dawla al-Marwāniyya* "the Marwānid dynasty" here refers more specifically to Marwān I ibn al-Ḥakam (reg. 64/684–65/685).

237 Ahrun ("Ἀῤῥων?) ibn Aʿyan was an Alexandrian presbyter (*qass*) who lived in the late 6th or early 7th century CE; he authored a voluminous medical 'Compendium' (*Σύνταγμα*?) which was subsequently translated from Greek into Syriac by a certain Gōsiōs (Gessius?), and eventually from Syriac into Arabic by Māsarjawayh (though the latter allegation is challenged by Ullmann [UllMed 23]); both the Greek and the Syriac versions of Ahrun's book are lost, but we possess a fair number of Arabic quotations from it (s.t. *Kunnāsh Ahrun*), see UllMed 87 ff. and GaS 3/166 ff.

238 Cf. note 233 above.

239 Read *arbaʿūna* (instead of *arbaʿīna*).

This story was told to me by Abū Bakr Muḥammad ibn ʿUmar ibn ʿAbd al-ʿAzīz,[240] in the mosque of Carmona,[241] in the year 359.[242]

﴿٦٣﴾ **The seventh generation:** sages of the Islamic Era who excelled at medicine and philosophy —some of them Muslims,[243] some Christians—

20
Bukhtīshūʿ[244]

the physician. He adhered to the Christian creed. He lived in the days of Abū l-ʿAbbās, the Commander of the Faithful and founder [of the ʿAbbāsid dynasty], whom he accompanied and whom he treated.[245] He was eminent in the art of medicine, and much revered throughout Baghdad for his knowledge and association with the caliph and his sons.

﴿٦٤﴾ 21
Jibrīl

ibn Bukhtīshūʿ,[246] a skilled [and] distinguished physician. Bukhtīshūʿ[247] wrote works on medicine, like his book [titled] *On Cosmetics*,[248] or like a *Small*

240 That is Ibn al-Qūṭiyya, a philologist and historian from Córdoba, who is best known for a work titled *Taʾrīkh iftitāḥ al-Andalus* "History of the Conquest of al-Andalus"; he died in the year 367/977, see BoViIḲ and MoIQ *passim*.

241 Arabic *al-Qarmūnā*, a town in southwestern Spain, about 20 miles east of Seville.

242 That is 970 CE.

243 The text here has اسلام, which is odd. It may be emended to *al-islām*, in the sense of *ahl al-islām* "the adherents of Islam" (cf. LaLex 1416c); or it may be read *aslām*, a broken plural of *silm* "he who keeps (or: is at) peace", and by extension "he who submits to Islam" (?).

244 Bukhtīshūʿ ibn Jurjīs, a Nestorian, was director of the hospital at Gondēshāpūr before the ʿAbbāsid caliph Hārūn al-Rashīd (reg. 170/786–193/809) summoned him to Baghdad (in 171/787), where he rose to be court physician; Bukhtīshūʿ died in the year 185/801, see UllMed 109 no. 2, GaS 3/210 f. and InkBu *passim*.

245 This is a chronological blunder: the caliph Abū l-ʿAbbās al-Saffāḥ (not *al-Qāʾim*) reigned from 132/750 to 136/754, decades before the arrival of Bukhtīshūʿ ibn Jurjīs in Baghdad; cf. also note 251 below.

246 Jibrīl ibn Bukhtīshūʿ was appointed court physician to Hārūn al-Rashīd in 190/805, and later also attended the caliphs al-Amīn and al-Maʾmūn, Hārūn's sons; Jibrīl died in the year 212/827 or 213/828, see UllMed 109 no. 3, GaS 3/226 f. and InkBu *passim*.

247 Here, the narrative returns, at least temporarily, to biography 20.

248 There is no other record to connect Bukhtīshūʿ ibn Jurjīs (or any member of his illustrious clan) with a writing on 'cosmetics' (*zīna*), presumably including dermatologic issues.

Compendium which is attributed to him.[249] He served [the caliph] al-Manṣūr bi-llāh;[250] then, having raised his son Jibrīl, [the latter] took his place, was just as high-minded as his father, and [in turn] rendered service to the ʿAbbāsid rulers.[251]

﴾٦٥﴿ 22
Yūḥannā ibn Māsawayh[252]

[He was] a Syrian Christian. [Hārūn] al-Rashīd entrusted him with the translation of ancient medical books which were found in Ancyra,[253] Amorium,[254] and [other] cities of the Byzantines captured by the Muslims; he appointed him as chief translator, and assigned to him [a number of] accomplished clerks to do the writing.[255] [Yūḥannā] served [the caliphs] Hārūn, al-Amīn and al-

249 This is almost certainly a reference to Bukhtīshūʿ ibn Jurjīs' medical handbook otherwise known as *Kunnāsh mukhtaṣar* "Concise Compendium" (here: *Kunnāsh ṣaghīr*); for (Arabic) quotations from presumably this text see UllMed 109 note 2 and GaS 3/211.

250 This is another chronological blunder (and self-contradiction) on the part of Ibn Juljul: the caliph Abū Jaʿfar al-Manṣūr bi-llāh reigned from 136/754 to 158/775, several years before Bukhtīshūʿ ibn Jurjīs arrived in Baghdad; cf. also the following note.

251 Looking back at biographies **20** and **21**, it is clear that Ibn Juljul's sources for the Bukhtīshūʿ family-of-physicians must have been rather shaky. It is certainly true that the first four members carry names which can easily be confused: Jurjīs ibn Jibrīl ibn Bukhtīshūʿ (d. after 151/768), father of Bukhtīshūʿ ibn Jurjīs (d. 185/801), father of Jibrīl ibn Bukhtīshūʿ (d. 212–213/827–828), father of Bukhtīshūʿ ibn Jibrīl (d. 256/870); and whilst Ibn Juljul rightly places his two protagonists in the early ʿAbbāsid period, he nonetheless mixes up the caliphs, naming Abū l-ʿAbbās (instead of Hārūn al-Rashīd) and al-Manṣūr (instead of Hārūn, al-Amīn and al-Maʾmūn). The work title *Fī l-Zīna* "On Cosmetics" appears out of nowhere, and its alleged author, Bukhtīshūʿ ibn Jurjīs, is said to have lived in the days of Abū l-ʿAbbās (**20**) but also to have served al-Manṣūr (**21**). On the other hand, the association of Bukhtīshūʿ ibn Jurjīs with a "Small Compendium"; the statement that he fathered Jibrīl; and the indication that the latter served several ʿAbbāsid caliphs—all these are sound items of information.

252 Abū Zakariyyāʾ Yūḥannā (sometimes Yaḥyā) ibn Māsawayh was born around the year 160/777 in Gondēshāpūr, into a family of Syrian Nestorian physicians; he came to Iraq with his father Abū Yūḥannā Māsawayh, and spent almost all his life as a hospital director and court physician to several ʿAbbāsid caliphs in Baghdad and Samarra; his organization of translations (from Greek and/or Syriac) has left no tangible trace, i.e. there are no extant texts of that kind connected to his name; Yūḥannā died in the year 243/857 in Samarra, see UllMed 112–115, GaS 3/231–236 and VaIM *passim*.

253 Arabic *Anqira* < *Ἄγκυρα*, a city in central Anatolia (today's Ankara).

254 Arabic *ʿAmmūriyya* < *Ἀμόριον*, an ancient city in central Anatolia.

255 Ancyra and Amorium were sacked by Muslim armies in the summer of 223/838, in the course of a major military campaign led by the then ʿAbbāsid caliph al-Muʿtaṣim (reg. 218/833–227/842); these events took place more than thirty years after the death of Hārūn

Ma'mūn, and he continued in that [service] until the days of al-Mutawakkil.[256] The Hāshimid rulers[257] would not eat any food unless he was present; he used to stand next to them with jars containing warm, cooked, digestive electuaries to strengthen the innate heat in winter, and with cooling beverages and pastes in summer. He was regarded with utmost respect in Baghdad and wielded considerable power.

His medical secrets he consigned, for the benefit of people, to [several writings]: a book which he called *The Proof*, in thirty chapters; [then] his book known as *The Insight*; his book known as *Completion and Completeness*; his book [titled] *On Fevers*; his book *On Bloodletting and Cupping*; his book *On Drugs*; his book known as ﴿٦٦﴾ *The Branched*, [which is] an extensive [medical] compendium; his book *On Leprosy*, the first of its kind; his book *On Foodstuffs*; his book on the stomach known as *The Sinking Scale*; or his book *On Purgative Drugs and their Administration*.[258] He authored many other writings

---

al-Rashīd, whom Ibn Juljul here wrongly associates with the translation of Greek books *that were brought back from this campaign*. In a more general sense, however, it seems that it was indeed Hārūn who first put Yūḥannā in charge of translating "ancient medical books", see BHDuw 227,10 f. (there, the link between this appointment and any books from Ancyra or Amorium is rightly missing).

256 The combined reign of Hārūn al-Rashīd, al-Amīn, al-Ma'mūn, *al-Muʿtaṣim*, *al-Wāthiq* and al-Mutawakkil stretches from 170/786 to 247/861; Yūḥannā would have been in his early twenties halfway through Hārūn's caliphate, and about seventy at the beginning of al-Mutawakkil's caliphate.

257 The Hāshimids (*Banū Hāshim*) are the ʿAbbāsids, who descended from *Hāshim* ibn ʿAbd Manāf, the great-grandfather of the prophet Muḥammad, through the latter's paternal uncle *al-ʿAbbās* ibn ʿAbd al-Muṭṭalib.

258 This is a somewhat random selection of Yūḥannā's writings. In the sequence given above by Ibn Juljul, the Arabic titles are: *al-Burhān* "The Proof" (medical philosophy?); *al-Baṣīra* "The Insight" (ophthalmology, cf. UllMed 205); *al-Kamāl wa-l-tamām* "Completion and Completeness" (general medicine, cf. UllMed 113); *Fī l-Ḥummayāt* "On Fevers"; *Fī l-Faṣd wa-l-ḥijāma* "On Bloodletting and Cupping"; *Fī l-Adwiya* "On Drugs"; *al-Mushajjar* "The Branched" (a medical compendium [*kunnāsh*] in the form of branch-diagrams, cf. UllMed 113); *Fī l-Judhām* "On Leprosy"; *Fī l-Aghdhiya* "On Foodstuffs"; *al-Rujḥān* "The Sinking Scale" (gastrology, perhaps dealing with excess weight, cf. IAU 3.1/486 no. 12); *Fī l-Adwiya al-mushila wa-iṣlāḥihā* "On Purgative Drugs and their Administration". Some of Yūḥannā's writings are preserved as manuscripts, few are edited, some are partially accessible through more or less extensive quotations, and some are only known by their titles, cf. UllMed 113 ff. and GaS 3/233–236; among the eleven writings listed by Ibn Juljul, we possess quotations from *al-Kamāl wa-l-tamām* (cf. GaS 3/235 no. 33), and manuscripts of *Fī l-Ḥummayāt*, *Fī l-Faṣd wa-l-ḥijāma*, *al-Mushajjar*, *Fī l-Judhām*, *Fī l-Aghdhiya* and *Fī l-Adwiya al-mushila wa-iṣlāḥihā* (cf. GaS 3/233 nos 2, 5, 7 and 235 nos 20, 22, 23); the title *Fī l-Adwiya* is up in the air.

on subjects that only he could have dealt with.[259] Ḥunayn ibn Isḥāq[260] was his pupil and servant. [Yūḥannā] was a physician who had a keen penchant for worded style[261] and [medical] treatment; he stands [proud] in the line of those [sages] that have gone before him.

﴾٦٧﴿ 23
Yūḥannā ibn al-Biṭrīq[262]

the translator, a client[263] of al-Ma'mūn, the Commander of the Faithful.[264] [Yūḥannā] was chief translator, [a task] which he accomplished [using] nice expressions though his Arabic was rather poor.[265] He translated a lot of the works of the ancients, [like] Aristotle's book for Alexander, which is known as *The Secret of Secrets* or else *The Policy of Good Government*.[266]

---

259 The most complete list of Yūḥannā's writings is given in GaS 3/233–236 (57 titles).

260 On Ḥunayn ibn Isḥāq see biography **24** below.

261 The Arabic term employed here by Ibn Juljul is *ta'līf*, lit. "putting (things) together, composing (a book)"; note that the lemma may also be read as a plural, scil. *ta'ālīf* (Arabic تاليف for both). I have translated it by "worded style", implying also a connotation of *spoken* style, on the grounds that Yūḥannā was known in particular for his scintillating wit and caustic humour, as is evidenced by various anecdotes in that vein, see e.g. IAU 3.1/466–485 (the latter, having spilled a lot of ink on circulating precisely such anecdotes, finishes by strongly disapproving of Yūḥannā's 'ungodly' mannerisms).

262 Yūḥannā (often Yaḥyā) ibn al-Biṭrīq was active as a translator and author in Baghdad around the end of the 2nd/8th and the beginning of the 3rd/9th centuries; his family traced back to the Christian population of North Africa who spoke 'African Latin' (*al-lisān al-laṭīnī al-ifrīqī*), which is why he is sometimes called a 'Latin' (*laṭīnī*), in the sense of 'speaker of vernacular Byzantine Greek' (IAU 3.1/549 with note 43); he was probably born in Iraq, because his father, al-Biṭrīq (Πατρίκιος), already worked as a translator for the 'Abbāsid caliph al-Manṣūr (reg. 136/754–158/775); Yūḥannā seems to have converted to Islam at some point, for Ibn Juljul subsequently describes him as a 'client' (*mawlan*, cf. the following note); the date of his death is not certain but sometimes given as 200/815, see UllMed 326, GaS 3/225 and StrIB *passim*.

263 The term *mawlan* "client" normally denotes the subordinate individual in the Arabo-Islamic patronage system. Generally speaking, a client may either be a freed slave whose former owner becomes his patron, or he may be a free non-Muslim (like Yūḥannā) who, upon conversion to Islam, enters into a binding relationship with a socially superior Arab Muslim patron, cf. NawCl *passim*.

264 The 'Abbāsid caliph al-Ma'mūn reigned from 198/813 to 218/833; if Yūḥannā died indeed "around 200/815" (GaS 3/225 and IAU 3.1/549 note 41), he must have become al-Ma'mūn's 'client' either before the latter acceded to the caliphate, or very shortly thereafter.

265 That is, he translated paraphrastically.

266 As no Greek (nor Syriac) text of this pseudo-Aristotelian writing is anywhere on record, the story of its 'translation' into Arabic is most probably a myth, cf. note 99 above; for Yūḥannā's *genuine* translations see DunTr 144ff.

Yūḥannā mentions that he went off to look for this [book], and that in his quest he visited [many] temples. Eventually he came to the Temple of Heliopolis,[267] which Hermes the Great[268] had built for himself to praise in it God the Sublime. [Yūḥannā then] says: "There at last I encountered an ascetic monk, a man of profound knowledge and deep insight, whom I befriended and beguiled until he gave me access to the books that were kept in the temple. Among them I found the object of my search, which the Commander of the Faithful[269] had instructed me to obtain; [it was] written in gold. And so I returned to the Victorious Majesty, possessing what had been desired".[270]

This Yūḥannā was not a physician, philosophy being his main concern; he served no king nor prince in a medical capacity.

﴿٦٨﴾ 24
Ḥunayn ibn Isḥāq[271]

the pupil of Yūḥannā ibn Māsawayh.[272] He knew the language of the Arabs, was highly proficient in the Greek language, and possessed such competence in both as to be able to discern their finest subtleties.[273] He set off from Baghdad for the land of Persia, ﴿٦٩﴾ where al-Khalīl ibn Aḥmad the grammarian lived[274]—may God have mercy upon him. Ḥunayn stayed with him until he had fully mastered the language of the Arabs, and he [subsequently] introduced the *Book of the* [*Letter*] *ʿAyn* to Baghdad.[275] Then he was chosen and

267 Read *ʿAyn* (instead of *ʿAbd* var. *ʿĪd*) *al-Shams* "Heliopolis".

268 Hermes the Great (*Hirmis al-akbar*) may be identical with Ibn Juljul's 'first' or, less likely, 'third' Hermes, cf. biographies 1 and 3 above.

269 That is the aforenamed caliph al-Maʾmūn, cf. note 264 above.

270 This enterprising story, which Ibn Juljul must have copied directly from Yūḥannā's introduction to the Arabic version of the *Secret of Secrets* (JulṬab 67 f. notes 4–11), is probably just as much of an invention as the translation itself, cf. DunTr 148.

271 Abū Zayd Ḥunayn ibn Isḥāq al-ʿIbādī was born in the year 192/808 in al-Ḥīra, southern Iraq, into a family of Nestorian Arabs; he is widely regarded as the most brilliant translator ever from Greek into Syriac and Arabic; he died in the year 260/873 or 264/877, probably in Baghdad or Samarra, see UllMed 115–119, GaS 3/247–256 and StrḤu *passim*.

272 On Yūḥannā ibn Māsawayh see biography 22 above.

273 Read *ʿalal*.

274 al-Khalīl ibn Aḥmad al-Farāhidī, a pioneering Arab philologist, was born in Oman, grew up in Basra, and died there in 175/791 (perhaps even a few years earlier and in any case before Ḥunayn was born). Ibn Juljul's assertion that Ḥunayn studied under al-Khalīl is therefore a chronological impossibility which could be interpreted as an attempt to link Ḥunayn's linguistic prowess to the founder of Arabic grammar; there is, by the way, no record to support the claim that al-Khalīl ever resided in Persia. On al-Khalīl see SellKh *passim*.

275 al-Khalīl is credited with the compilation of the first Arabic dictionary, titled *Kitāb al-*

commissioned to translate. The one who selected him for this [task] was Jaʿfar al-Mutawakkil ʿalā llāh;[276] he [also] assigned to him [a number of] skilled, experienced translator-clerks who produced [draft] versions which Ḥunayn revised. Among [these translator-clerks] were Isṭīfan ibn Basīl,[277] Ḥubaysh,[278] Mūsā ibn Khālid the translator,[279] and Yaḥyā ibn Hārūn.[280]

Ḥunayn rendered medical service to al-Mutawakkil ʿalā llāh.[281] He always wore a waist-belt which designated him as a Christian.[282] He learned the Greek language in Alexandria.[283] He was a magnificent translator—it was he who

---

ʿAyn "Book of the (Letter) *ʿAyn*", which is arranged (probably under Indian influence), not alphabetically but according to groups of sounds or points of articulation, beginning with the letter-phoneme *ʿayn* (ع).

276 That is the tenth ʿAbbāsid caliph Jaʿfar ibn Muḥammad al-Mutawakkil ʿalā llāh (reg. 232/847–247/861).

277 Isṭīfan ibn Basīl (Στέφανος ὁ τοῦ Βασιλείου), an ethnic Greek, is known to have translated several Galenic works into Arabic; his main achievement, however, was a translation of Dioscorides' *Περὶ ὕλης ἰατρικῆς* (Latin *De materia medica*), which he accomplished around the middle of the 3rd/9th century in Baghdad; Ḥunayn *sometimes* revised Isṭīfan's translations. See UllMM 21–24; further UllMed 259 f. and GaS 3/58 ff.

278 Ḥubaysh ibn al-Ḥasan al-Aʿsam (fl. second half of 3rd/9th century) was a nephew and pupil of Ḥunayn, with whom he collaborated on the translation of Greek works into Syriac and Arabic, see UllMed 119, GaS 3/265 f. and StrḤub *passim*.

279 Mūsā ibn (not: ibn *Abī*) Khālid 'the translator' (*al-tarjumān*) is a somewhat obscure personality: Ibn Abī Uṣaybiʿa (d. 668/1270), who copied Ibn Juljul's above account more or less literally (IAU 3.1/503), makes the isolated claim, elsewhere in his book, that Mūsā ibn Khālid translated, inter alia, Galen's *Summaria* (cf. note 172 above) into Arabic, see op.cit. 3.1/546—there, the editorial assertion in note 23 that Mūsā was a disciple of Ḥunayn represents a circular (and hence futile) conclusion, because it is drawn from another 7th/13th century source that itself merely reiterates Ibn Juljul's account. An older source, Ibn al-Nadīm's (d. 380/990) *Catalogue*, intriguingly registers a certain Mūsā ibn Khālid in a list of early 'transmitters/translators' (*naqala*) from Persian (!) into Arabic, see NadFih 1/244,27.

280 The reading Yaḥyā ibn Hārūn is an editorial emendation obtained from QifTaʾ 171,11 (Ibn Juljul's text originally reads *Yaḥyā al-Naḥwī* [crossed out in the base manuscript, cf. JulṬab 71 note 8], scil. John the Grammarian, which is chronologically impossible).

281 Cf. note 276 above. The editor of Ibn Juljul's text here implants, for no apparent reason, a phrase which he obtained from a parallel passage in Ibn Abī Uṣaybiʿa's history (IAU 3.1/503,18 f.), namely: "during which time he [Ḥunayn] enjoyed a tenure of good graces" (*wa-ḥaẓiya fī ayyāmihī*).

282 *zunnār* denotes "the *thing which the free non-Muslim subject of a Muslim government, who pays a poll-tax for his freedom and toleration*, i.e. [a] Christian, Jew or Sabian, *binds upon his waist*" (LaLex 1258c); the term is derived from *ζωνάριον*, dim. of *ζώνη* "belt, girdle" (LSLex 637b).

283 It is, in fact, not entirely clear where Ḥunayn learned Greek. Having fallen out with his teacher Yūḥannā ibn Māsawayh, he 'disappeared' for two years into the Byzantine realm and returned with Homeric poetry on his lips; the current consensus seems to be that he stayed in Constantinople, see StrḤu *passim*.

elucidated the expressions in the books of Hippocrates and Galen, prepared wonderful summaries of those [works], shed light on difficult passages in them, and resolved their problematic aspects. He [also] authored a number of outstandingly erudite[284] and useful writings. His approach to the works of Galen was modelled on that of the Alexandrians: he recast them into question-and-answer form, and he did that really well.

His is a book [titled] *On the Art of Logic*, unsurpassed in its clear arrangement and skillful organization; he [also] wrote a splendid book [titled] *On Foodstuffs*; his is a book [titled] *On Regimen for Convalescents* and [another] *On Laxative Remedies and Foodstuffs in Health Regimen*, the first of its kind; he [moreover] authored a *Compendium* which he condensed from the book of Paulus.[285] [Ḥunayn's] writings are numerous,[286] and if it were less long-winded I would name them all.

[Ḥunayn] begot two sons: Dāwud and Isḥāq. As regards Isḥāq, he followed his [father] in translating [Greek works], which [task] he accomplished with perfect mastery; for his part, he was strongly drawn to philosophy, and he translated Aristotle the philosopher's book [*On*] *the Soul*, in seven treatises, which he found with the commentary of Themistios.[287] As for Dāwud, he was a physician.[288]

---

284 Read *mutqana*.

285 As Ibn Juljul indicates himself at the end of this paragraph, the present list of titles offers just a small selection. In the given sequence, the Arabic equivalents are: *Fī Ṣināʿat al-manṭiq* (lost, authentic?); *Fī l-Aghdhiya* (preserved, see UllMed 199 and GaS 3/253 no. 5); *Fī Tadbīr al-nāqihīna* (preserved, see UllMed 117 [*-nāqih*] and GaS 3/255 no. 10 [read *-nāqih* instead of *-nāqa*!]); *Fī l-Adwiya al-mushila wa-l-aghdhiya ʿalā tadbīr al-ṣiḥḥa* (perhaps identical with the [lost] *Tadbīr al-aṣiḥḥāʾ bi-l-maṭʿam wa-l-mashrab*, cited UllMed 199); the abridged *Kunnāsh* which Ḥunayn allegedly composed on the basis of the compendium of *Būlush* (*Παῦλος*) is most probably connected to Paul of Aegina's (fl. 7th century CE) *Πραγματεία*, a medical handbook in *seven* parts and hence known in Arabic as *Kunnāsh al-Thurayyā* "Compendium of the Pleiades", cf. UllMed 86 f. with PorPP 7 f. and *passim* (where Ḥunayn frequently figures as the *translator* of Paul's work, e.g. 47 f., 111 ff. and 220 f.).

286 IAU 3.1/521–531: 111 titles; cf. GaS 3/249–256.

287 Isḥāq ibn Ḥunayn (d. 298/910) translated, inter alia, nearly all texts of the Aristotelian corpus into Arabic, including the abovementioned *Περὶ ψυχῆς* "On the Soul" (Arabic *Fī l-Nafs*, here: *Kitāb al-Nafs*), see StrIḤ *passim*. Themistios (Arabic *Thāmisṭiyūs* < *Θεμίστιος*) was a philosopher and politician, known mainly for his paraphrases and epitomes of Aristotelian writings, including *Περὶ ψυχῆς*; he died in 385 CE.

288 Dāwud ibn Ḥunayn is hardly known. Ibn Abī Uṣaybiʿa confirms that Dāwud was a physician (of sorts), and that he left no written works apart from a single 'Compendium' (*Kunnāsh*), see IAU 3.1/501,17–20. Note in passing that Ḥunayn must have had a third son, as he is also called *Abū Zayd*.

Ḥunayn died of grief one night. I will now relate an interesting story about this, which I was told by the vizier of[289] al-Ḥakam al-Mustanṣir bi-llāh, the Commander of the Faithful.[290] [This vizier] said: "We were[291] in the company of the Commander of the Faithful, al-Mustanṣir bi-llāh—may God be pleased with him. The conversation was flowing, when he said: 'Do you know the circumstances around the death of Ḥunayn ibn Isḥāq?' [As] we replied 'No, O Commander of the Faithful', he said: '[It was that] al-Mutawakkil ʿalā llāh[292] went out one day, suffering from a hangover, and sat down in ﴾٧٠﴿ his [usual] place, exposed to the sun. With him were the Christian physician[293] al-Ṭayfūrī[294] and Ḥunayn ibn Isḥāq. [When] al-Ṭayfūrī remarked: «O Commander of the Faithful! The sun is harmful for a hangover», al-Mutawakkil said to Ḥunayn: «What is your opinion on that?» Ḥunayn ibn Isḥāq replied: «O Commander of the Faithful! The sun is not harmful for a hangover». And as the two [physicians] started to argue with each other in front of him, [the caliph] demanded that both demonstrate the soundness of their [respective] statements. Ḥunayn said: «O Commander of the Faithful! A hangover is the condition of the person who suffers from it—the sun does not harm the hangover but the person who has it». al-Mutawakkil exclaimed: «Ḥunayn wins, for he clearly understands the nature of words and the definition of expressions better than his colleagues!», and al-Ṭayfūrī was left speechless. Later on the same day, [when] Ḥunayn took out from his sleeve a book[295] in which there was an illustration of Christ on the cross, surrounded by a number of Jews, al-

---

289 In the given context, the preposition *ʿan* makes no sense and should have been discarded by the editor of the text; accordingly, *wazīrun* (*sic*) is to be read *wazīru*.

290 That is the second Umayyad caliph of Córdoba, al-Ḥakam II ibn ʿAbd al-Raḥmān al-Mustanṣir bi-llāh (reg. 350/961–366/976); the vizier referred to here is probably Jaʿfar ibn ʿUthmān al-Muṣḥafī (d. 372/982), cf. FagBM 2/391, 413ff., 420f. and *passim* with LéP-rEM 109.

291 Better read *kunnā* (instead of *kuntu*).

292 Cf. note 276 above.

293 Read with IAU 2.1/475,-4: *al-ṭabīb* (instead of *al-kātib* "the clerk").

294 Isrāʾīl ibn Zakariyyāʾ al-Ṭayfūrī (fl. mid 3rd/9th century) was the personal physician of al-Fatḥ ibn Khāqān; the latter, erstwhile captain of the palace guard and later, under al-Mutawakkil, holder of various high government offices, belonged to the innermost circle of power. This explains Ibn Abī Uṣaybiʿa's remark that al-Ṭayfūrī, by extension, occupied an "unassailable position" (*manzila makīna*) in the caliph's entourage (IAU 3.1/418), and it also goes a long way to explain the outcome of the story at hand.

295 In Ibn Abī Uṣaybiʿa's account, at least according to some manuscripts, the subject of this sentence is not Ḥunayn but al-Ṭayfūrī, i.e. "he [al-Ṭayfūrī] took out from his sleeve a book [to show] to (*li-*) Ḥunayn" (IAU 2.1/476,1 [adopted by the editors 3.1/506,-11]); this variant does, in fact, make more sense, but as Ibn Juljul's reading is confirmed by al-Qifṭī (QifTaʾ 172,11), we have not emended it.

Ṭayfūrī said to him: «O Ḥunayn! Are those [the people] who crucified Christ?» [When Ḥunayn] answered «Yes», al-Ṭayfūrī said to him: «Spit on them, then!» [And when] Ḥunayn replied «No, I will not!» and al-Ṭayfūrī asked «Why not?», Ḥunayn said: «Because they are not really [the people] who crucified Christ—these are just drawings». This [reply] infuriated[296] al-Ṭayfūrī and he got up to [see] al-Mutawakkil, whom he asked for his permission to let a Christian jury pass judgement on [Ḥunayn]. An envoy was sent to[297] the Catholicos and [his] bishops who, when the question was posed to them, responded with the excommunication of Ḥunayn—seventy times he was cursed in the presence of the Christian congregation, and his waist-belt was cut off. [For his part] al-Mutawakkil ordered that [henceforth] no medicine prescribed by Ḥunayn must be presented to him unless al-Ṭayfūrī had watched over its preparation. Ḥunayn departed to his house and died that very night. It is said that he died of grief,[298] or that he made himself swallow poison'". And this is the story of Ḥunayn ibn Isḥāq the translator's death.

﴿٧٣﴾ 25
Abū Yūsuf Yaʿqūb ibn Isḥāq

ibn al-Ṣabbāḥ al-Kindī,[299] a Basran[300] of noble stock whose grandfather had been a provincial governor for the Hāshimids.[301] [al-Kindī] left Basra and the estate he possessed there, and moved to Baghdad where he refined his education.

He was learned in medicine, philosophy, arithmetic, logic, musical composition, geometry, numerology, astronomy and astrology. No other philosopher of Islam followed in his writings the example of Aristotle as much as he did. He [produced] numerous works on [various] branches of science.[302] He put him-

296 Read *fa-'shtadda* (instead of *fa-ashhada*).

297 Read *ilā* (instead of *fī*).

298 The editorial addition of *wa-asafan* "and of sorrow" (obtained from IAU 2.1/476,7) is unnecessary.

299 That is the famous 'philosopher of the Arabs' (d. ca. 256/870), a true polymath, extremely versatile scientist and remarkably prolific writer, on whom see JRKin and AdKin *passim*; further UllMed 123 (medicine) and 301f. (pharmacy) with GaS 3/244–247 (medicine) and 375f. (zoology).

300 The view apparently held by most later Arab authors is that al-Kindī hailed from Kufa (not Basra), cf. JulṬab 73 ad 25.

301 The Hāshimids (*Banū Hāshim*) are the ʿAbbāsids, and in the present context the *early* ʿAbbāsids; cf. also note 257 above.

302 IAU 3.1/567(with note 95)–587: 283 titles.

self at the service of rulers whose cultural interests he nourished. He translated a lot of [Greek] philosophical texts,[303] elucidating difficulties, ﴿٧٤﴾ summarizing complexities, and simplifying obscurities. His is a book on monotheism, [written] in the manner of the logicians [and titled] *On the Procedural Steps towards Demonstration*,[304] the first of its kind; a book [titled] *On the Affirmation of Prophethood*,[305] [written] in the same style; he [authored] a book which he called *The Path to Virtues in the Cultivation of the Soul*;[306] [further] a book about geography [titled] *On the Knowledge of Inhabited Climes*,[307] as well as others [in that vein]; and [there is a book titled] *Solving Riddles*.[308]

﴿٧٥﴾ 26
Thābit ibn Qurra al-Ḥarrānī[309]

He resided in the city of Baghdad. Philosophy, more than medicine, was his main concern. He lived during the reign of al-Muʿtaḍid.[310] He [wrote] many

303 Whether al-Kindī himself actually *translated* Greek works is a matter of dispute—he was no doubt involved as a well-placed advocate, mentor and possibly even sponsor of such translations, but apart from that, his role seems to have largely consisted in the stylistic revision of certain Arabic translations, in the 'correction' of draft renditions, and perhaps in some paraphrastic recasts of Greek philosophical texts, see AdKin *passim*.

304 *Fī Sulūk marātib al-burhān*, not attested elsewhere.

305 *Fī Ithbāt al-nubuwwa* (so also ṢAṬab 52,9), otherwise known as *Fī Tathbīt al-rusul—ʿalayhim al-salām* "On the Affirmation of the Prophets—peace be upon them", see NadFih 1/259,14 f.; QifTa' 373,10 f.; IAU 3.1/579 no. 175.

306 *Sabīl al-faḍāʾil fī ādāb al-nafs*. The first part of this title appears elsewhere as *Tashīl subul al-faḍāʾil* "On Facilitating the Paths to Virtues", see NadFih 1/260,2; QifTa' 374,4; IAU 3.1/581 no. 198. The second part is not, as Ibn Juljul has it, an extension of the first but rather a separate title, viz. *Ādāb al-nafs* "The Cultivation of the Soul", see ṢAṬab 52,10.

307 *Fī Maʿrifat al-aqālīm al-maʿmūra*, not attested elsewhere. Note, however, that al-Qifṭī (QifTa' 98,14 f.) registers, in his bibliography of Claudius Ptolemy, a work titled *The Geography of the Inhabited Earth* (i.q. *Γεωγραφικὴ ὑφήγησις*?), which he says "was nicely translated (!) into Arabic by al-Kindī" (*naqalahu l-Kindī ilā l-ʿarabī naql*[an] *jayyid*[an]).

308 *Istikhrāj al-muʿammā*, perhaps identical with *Fī l-Asmāʾ al-muʿammāh* "On Riddling Names", see NadFih 1/261,8; QifTa' 375,16 f.; IAU 3.1/585 no. 254.

309 Abū l-Ḥasan Thābit ibn Qurra al-Ḥarrānī, a Sabian by religion, was born around the year 211/826 in Ḥarrān, an ancient city in Upper Mesopotamia, where he worked as a money-changer before moving to Baghdad; famed primarily as a mathematician, he wrote original works on a great variety of subjects; trilingual (Greek-Syriac-Arabic), he initially translated texts and/or revised existing translations for the Banū Mūsā; later in life, he became court astronomer of the caliph al-Muʿtaḍid (cf. the following note); Thābit died in the year 288/901, see RMThā *passim*; further the literature cited IAU 3.1/593 note 1 (adding UllMed 123 f. [medicine]).

310 That is the sixteenth ʿAbbāsid caliph Aḥmad ibn Ṭalḥa al-Muʿtaḍid bi-llāh (reg. 279/892–289/902); the reading *al-Muʿtaḍid* is a justified editorial emendation obtained from QifTa'

books on [different] branches of science,[311] like logic, arithmetic, geometry, astrology and astronomy; [among them] is a wonderful work [titled] *Introduction to the Book of Euclid*.[312] In terms of [scientific] knowledge, [Thābit] stands proud in the line of [his] predecessors.

﴾٧٦﴿ 27
Qusṭā ibn Lūqā al-Baʿlabakkī[313]

[He was] a Christian by faith, a skilled, high-minded physician, a philosopher [and] an astrologer, learned [also] in geometry and arithmetic. He [wrote] splendid works on medicine,[314] like his book [titled] *On the Predominance of Blood*,[315] or his book *On the Proportion of [Humoral] Mixtures*,[316] or his book *On the Difference between Soul and Spirit*,[317] or his book *On the Difference between Sound-Producing and Silent Animals*.[318] [Qusṭā] lived in the days of al-Muqtadir bi-llāh.[319]

115,10 f. (Ibn Juljul's original text erroneously has *al-Muqtadir*, whose reign only began seven years after Thābit's death). ŶulGen 74,-6 is to be emended accordingly.

311 IAU 3.1/600(with note 41)–610: 153 titles.

312 *Mudkhal ilā kitāb Uqlīdis*, referring to Euclid's (fl. 300 BCE) *Στοιχεῖα* or "Elements".

313 Qusṭā ibn Lūqā, a Melkite physician, scientist and translator (Greek-Syriac-Arabic), was born around the year 205/820 in the Levantine city of Baalbek; he travelled in Asia Minor before settling down in Baghdad; towards the end of his long life, following an invitation of the prince Sanḥārīb, he moved to Armenia, where he died in the year 300/912 (not "hacia el 288/900" [ŶulGen 120 note 102]), see UllMed 126, GaS 3/270 and HiḴL *passim*.

314 GaS 3/270–274: 51 (possibly 54) medical titles; cf. IAU 3.1/673–677 (62 titles, covering also non-medical topics).

315 *Fī Ghalabat al-dam*, otherwise known as *ʿIlal al-dam* "Blood Disorders" (implying a possible mix-up of غلبة / علل) or simply as *Kitāb/Maqāla fī l-Dam* "Book/Treatise on Blood", which forms part of a larger tetralogy on the constitution of the humours, see UllMed 126 and GaS 3/272 no. 18.

316 *Fī Nisbat al-akhlāṭ*, otherwise known as *Istiḥālat al-akhlāṭ* "The Alteration of (Humoral) Mixtures" and perhaps identical with the *Kitāb fī l-Akhlāṭ al-arbaʿa wa-mā tashtariku fīhī* "Book on the Four (Humoral) Mixtures and their Cooperation", see UllMed 126 and GaS 3/272 no. 25.

317 *Fī l-Farq* (var. *Faṣl*) *bayna l-nafs wa-l-rūḥ*, see UllMed 128.

318 *Fī l-Farq bayna l-ḥayawān al-nāṭiq wa-l-ṣāmit*; the title reappears IAU 3.1/675 no. 24 with the variation … *al-nāṭiq wa-ghayr al-nāṭiq*, translated by the editors as "… rational and non-rational animals", which is a perfectly legitimate rendition of the Arabic phrase but does, of course, imply something entirely different from Ibn Juljul's wording. ŶulGen 75,9 f. translates similarly "… el animal racional e irracional".

319 That is the eighteenth ʿAbbāsid caliph Jaʿfar ibn Aḥmad al-Muqtadir bi-llāh (reg. 295/908–320/932). Ibn Juljul's dating is correct only insofar as it refers to the tail-end of Qusṭā's life, which coincided with the childhood, adolescence and early reign of al-Muqtadir. Cf., however, JulṬab 76 note 3 and ŶulGen 120 note 103, where the emendation *al-Muʿtamid* is suggested.

﴿٧٧﴾ 28
Muḥammad ibn Zakariyyā' al-Rāzī[320]

[He was] a Muslim by faith, a man of culture [and] a clinical physician. He was in charge of the hospital of Rayy, then the hospital of Baghdad for some time.[321] Initially, he concentrated on playing the lute, then gave it up and devoted himself to the study of medicine and philosophy, in which two [fields] he reached the heights of [his] predecessors. He wrote many original works on medicine,[322] among them: his book which he called *The Collector*, in seventy treatises;[323] his book which he sent to al-Manṣūr ibn Khāqān;[324] his book which he called *The Poles*;[325] his book for 'Alī ibn Wahshūdhān, the governor of Tabaristan, which he called *Royal Medicine*;[326] his book [titled] *Dividing and Formgiving*;[327] his book *On Hamlets*[328] *and Villages*;[329] his book *On Spiritual*

---

320 Abū Bakr Muḥammad ibn Zakariyyā' al-Rāzī (latinized *Rhazes*) was born in the ancient Iranian city of Rayy in the year 251/865; he ranks among the most versatile and most authoritative physicians and thinkers in the history of Islam, exercising considerable influence on the subsequent course of medicine, alchemy and philosophy, also in the Latin West; he spent much of his adult life in Baghdad before finally returning to his birthplace Rayy, where he died in the year 313/925, see GoRā *passim* and KaCB 1f. with note 24.

321 It is fair to assume that Rayy, at the time, possessed no more than one hospital. As regards Baghdad, it had, when al-Rāzī arrived there around the year 284/897, also only one such institution, the so-called *Barāmika* (later simply *Old*) hospital; however, a second hospital, whose most propitious location al-Rāzī helped to determine and which became known as *Mu'taḍidī*, was built about three years later; another four hospitals were founded in quick succession between the years 301/914 and 313/925. It seems likely that the hospital which al-Rāzī is said to have directed was either the *Barāmika* or the *Mu'taḍidī* hospital, possibly even both; for further details see KaCB 2 note 27.

322 GaS 3/278–294: 143 medical titles.

323 *al-Jāmi'*, a compendious medical encyclopedia in *twelve sections* (IAU 3.2/862f. no. 92), perhaps identical with *al-Ḥāwī* "The Container", see UllMed 131, GaS 3/280f. and SSWF *passim*.

324 This is a reference to the so-called *(al-)Kitāb al-Manṣūrī* "Book for Manṣūr", which al-Rāzī composed in 290/903 and dedicated to the Sāmānid prince Abū Ṣāliḥ Manṣūr ibn Isḥāq, who at the time was governor of Rayy, see UllMed 132, GaS 3/281ff. no. 2 and BoAṢM *passim*. It is not clear wherefrom Ibn Juljul derived the designation "ibn *Khāqān*".

325 *al-Aqṭāb*, cf. also QifTa' 272,10.

326 *al-Ṭibb al-mulūkī*, dedicated to 'Alī ibn Wahshūdhān (Persian *Vahsudān*), the Jostanid governor of Rayy (not Tabaristan) from 299/912 to 303/916, see UllMed 133, GaS 3/286 no. 16 and PeJos *passim*.

327 *al-Taqsīm wa-l-tajsīd*, the latter term usually *tashjīr* "branching" (Arabic تشجير / تجسيد [metathesis?]), a nosological work in the form of branch diagrams, see UllMed 132 and GaS 3/284 no. 5.

328 Read *al-qurā* (instead of *al-quwā* [Arabic القوى / القرى]).

329 *Fī l-Qurā wa-l-dasākir*, var. *Fī l-Dasākīr wa-l-'izal* "On Villages and Counties", see QifTa' 272,12.

Medicine;[330] his book *On Gout*;[331] his book *On Smallpox*;[332] his book known as *Aphorisms*;[333] regarding Hippocrates and Galen, he wrote a book which he called *Doubts*;[334] he investigated the art of alchemy and wrote ﴿٧٨﴾ fourteen treatises about it;[335] and he wrote a book on bonesetting and dislocation.[336] Towards the end of his life he became blind, due to liquid descending into his eyes;[337] it was suggested to him that he could undergo couching, but he said: "No, I have seen enough of the world to be tired [of it]", and he would not allow his eyes to be couched. He lived during the reign of al-Muktafī.[338]

﴿٨٠﴾ 29
Thābit ibn Sinān ibn Thābit ibn Qurra the Sabian[339]

He lived in the days of al-Muṭīʿ li-llāh[340] and during the emirate of Aḥmad ibn Būyah 'the Amputee'.[341] Aḥmad ibn Yūnus al-Ḥarrānī,[342] in the course of his journey, met [Thābit] in Baghdad and studied under him—he told me so himself. [Thābit] was skilled in medicine, knowledgeable about its foundations, and good at unravelling [difficult] books.

---

330 *Fī l-Ṭibb al-rūḥānī*, see UllMed 136.

331 *Fī l-Niqris*, see GaS 3/288 no. 28 (s.t. *Awjāʿ al-niqris* "The Pains of Gout").

332 *Fī l-Judarī*, full title … *wa-l-ḥaṣba* "and measles", see UllMed 133 f. and GaS 3/283 no. 3.

333 *al-Fuṣūl*, also known as *al-Murshid* "The Guide", a didactic work on theoretical medicine inspired by Hippocrates' Ἀφορισμοί, see UllMed 134 f. and GaS 3/284 no. 7.

334 *al-Shukūk*, full title … *ʿalā Jālīnūs* "about Galen" (not Hippocrates), see UllMed 67 and GaS 3/77.

335 For al-Rāzī's alchemical works see e.g. RuBīr 47; it is quite possible that Ibn Juljul here alludes to al-Rāzī's main work on alchemy (*ṣanʿa*), which comprised of *twelve sections*, together with his *Kitāb al-Asrār* "Book of Secrets" and *Sirr al-asrār* "The Secret of Secrets", cf. IAU 3.2/856 f. nos 22, 25 and 26.

336 This seems to be a reference to al-Rāzī's *Risāla fī l-Jabr* "Epistle on Bonesetting", see GaS 3/293,-6 f.

337 That is, cataracts.

338 That is the seventeenth ʿAbbāsid caliph ʿAlī ibn Aḥmad al-Muktafī bi-llāh (reg. 289/902–295/908).

339 A physician, hospital director in Baghdad, author of a (lost) 'Chronicle' (*Taʾrīkh*), and grandson of Thābit ibn Qurra al-Ḥarrānī (on whom see biography 26 above); Thābit ibn Sinān died in the year 363/974 (IAU 3.1/623,11) or 365/976 (NadFih 1/302,25 f. and QifTaʾ 111,7–10).

340 That is the twenty-third ʿAbbāsid caliph al-Faḍl ibn al-Muqtadir al-Muṭīʿ li-llāh (reg. 334/946–363/974).

341 Aḥmad ibn Būyah Muʿizz al-Dawla (d. 356/967), the founder of Būyid supremacy in Iraq, was the *de facto* ruler of Baghdad from 334/946 up until his death; he owed his nickname *al-Aqṭaʿ* "the Amputee" to having lost a hand in battle. On him see ZeBuMD *passim*.

342 On Aḥmad ibn Yūnus, an older contemporary of Ibn Juljul, see biography 55/56 below.

﴿٨١﴾ 30
Ibn Waṣīf the Sabian[343]

Aḥmad ibn Yūnus al-Ḥarrānī[344] met him in Baghdad. [Ibn Waṣīf] was a physician, specialized in the treatment of the eye—nobody in his time knew more [about this subject] than he did.

[The following story] I was told by Aḥmad ibn Yūnus. He said: "I was in the presence of Ibn Waṣīf, who had lined up seven people to couch their eyes. Among them was a man, a native of Khorasan, whom he made to sit in front of him while he inspected his eyes. He saw liquid in them, indicating [the need for] couching. He named a fee, which was questioned, and so he agreed [to accept] eighty silver dirhams from the man, who swore that this was all he had. ﴿٨٢﴾ Persuaded, [Ibn Waṣīf] was about to draw [the man] closer to himself when his hand touched upon the latter's upper arm, where he discovered a small belt containing gold dinars. 'What is this?' asked Ibn Waṣīf. [When] the man from Khorasan squirmed, Ibn Waṣīf said: 'You falsely swear by God and yet hope that your eyesight will be restored? I, by God, shall not treat you, for you tried to deceive your Lord!' [The man] begged, but [Ibn Waṣīf] refused to couch him—he returned to him the eighty silver dirhams without couching his eyes".

31
Nasṭās[345]

He was an Egyptian and a Christian who lived during the reign of the Ikhshīdids.[346] An experienced physician, he was [particularly] good at uroscopy. He [wrote] an epistle[347] for the Andalusian Christian Yazīd ibn Rūmān,

---

343 *Aḥmad* (IAU 3.1/631,9) ibn Waṣīf was an oculist (*kaḥḥāl* [QifṬa' 395,19]) who practised in Baghdad around the middle of the 4th/10th century, cf. QifṬa' 436 and IAU 3.1/631 with note 1; it is possible, though by no means certain, that this Ibn Waṣīf is identical with *Ibrāhīm* ibn Waṣīf (Shāh) aka al-Waṣīfī, a much quoted authority on the history of ancient Egypt, see for a discussion SezWa *passim*. Note that Ibn Juljul's text erroneously reads *al-Ṣārī* (instead of *al-Ṣābiʾ* "the Sabian").

344 On Aḥmad ibn Yūnus, an older contemporary of Ibn Juljul, see biography 55/56 below.

345 Nasṭās (Ἀναστάσιος) ibn Jurayj, a Copt who was active before and around the middle of the 4th/10th century, see UllMed 138 and GaS 3/303.

346 The Ikhshīdid dynasty (read *al-Ikhshīd* instead of *al-Akhshīdh*) ruled Egypt and the western Levant from 323/935 to 358/969; according to QifṬa' 337,6f. and IAU 3.2/1147, Nasṭās lived more precisely under the *first* Ikhshīdid ruler, Muḥammad ibn Ṭughj (reg. 323/935–334/946).

347 Read with JulṬab 96,6: *risāla* (instead of *rasāʾil* "epistles").

[titled] *On Urine*;[348] he [also wrote] a splendid *Medical Compendium*.[349] He was very knowledgeable indeed.

﴿٨٤﴾ The **eighth generation**: sages of the Islamic Era who lived in the Maghreb

The first of them is

32
Isḥāq ibn ʿImrān nicknamed ʿInstant Poison'[350]

[He was] a Muslim by faith [and] originally from Baghdad. He came to Kairouan during the reign of Ziyādatallāh Ibn al-Aghlab.[351] [When] the latter sent for him, [Isḥāq] imposed three conditions, of which one remained unfulfilled:[352] upon his arrival, [Ibn al-Aghlab] was to dispatch a saddled camel to carry him; [provide him with] one thousand gold dinars to cover his expenses; and [write] a letter of safe-conduct in his own hand, ﴿٨٥﴾ so that he could return to his homeland whenever he wanted. Thanks to [Isḥāq], medicine arose in the Maghreb, and philosophy became known.[353] He was an able physician, distinguished [for his skill] in putting together compound drugs, well acquainted with the differentiation of diseases, and matching the ancients in terms of knowledge and ample talent. He settled in Kairouan for some time and composed [a number of] writings, among them: his book known as *The Diversion of*

348 *Fī l-Bawl* (preserved under the full title *Risāla fī Kayfiyyat al-istidlāl bi-l-bawl ʿalā aḥwāl al-shakhṣ wa-amrāḍihī* "Epistle on how to Deduce the Conditions of a Person and his Illnesses from the Urine", see GaS 3/303 no. 1). Note that in biography **38**, Ibn Juljul deals with a Christian physician from Córdoba named Khālid ibn Yazīd ibn Rūmān, saying that *he* was the addressee of Nasṭās' epistle, see JulṬab 96,5f.—this means that the above form of the name ought to be extended to *Khālid ibn* Yazīd …; according to GaS 3/303, this Khālid wrote, in turn, an epistle on 'Herbal Drugs' (*Adwiya shajariyya*) for Nasṭās.

349 *Kunnāsh fī l-ṭibb* (preserved, see GaS 3/303 no. 2).

350 Isḥāq ibn ʿImrān, a physician who died shortly before the year 296/909, see UllMed 125f. and GaS 3/266f.; according to IAU 3.2/999, he owed his nickname *Samm Sāʿa* 'Instant Poison' to the fact that "for all his knowledge, he was frequently unsuccessful in his treatment, and those who made use of his services died" (translation I. Sánchez).

351 That is the eleventh and last Aghlabid ruler of central North Africa (*Ifrīqiya*), Abū Muḍar Ziyādatallāh III ibn ʿAbdallāh ibn Ibrāhīm Ibn al-Aghlab (reg. 290/903–296/909).

352 The story soon to be told will clarify this 'unfulfilled condition' (*lam yafi lahū bi-aḥadihā*).

353 Read *ʿurifat*.

the Soul;[354] his book on the illness [called] melancholia,[355] unprecedented;[356] his book [titled] *On Bloodletting*;[357] or his book *On the Pulse*.[358] Over time, [Isḥāq] found it difficult to deal with Ziyādatallāh Ibn al-Aghlab, which led to such an estrangement between the two [men] that in the end Ibn al-Aghlab had him crucified.

[What happened was that] Isḥāq had asked for permission to return to Baghdad, which [Ibn al-Aghlab] did not grant. [Also] Isḥāq used to watch over Ibn al-Aghlab's food and say to him: "Eat this, omit that!", until [one day] a young Jew from al-Andalus was received by Ibn al-Aghlab and invited to join him, which he swiftly accepted and thereby became a witness to his meals; when Isḥāq said: "Leave this, do not eat it!", the Israelite remarked: "We would let you have it". [Moreover] Ibn al-Aghlab suffered from a respiratory disease, meaning [he was] short of breath. [On one occasion] curdled milk was put in front of him, which he intended to eat, but Isḥāq forbade it whilst the Israelite saw no harm and encouraged him to have it. In the night, [Ibn al-Aghlab] had so much difficulty breathing that he came close to death. [When] Isḥāq was called upon and asked: "Do you have any remedy?", he replied: "I forbade [curdled milk] but he did not follow my advice. I have no remedy". [The attendants] said to Isḥāq: "Here are five hundred gold dinars, now treat [him]!", yet he refused until [the sum] had reached one thousand *mithqāl*.[359] These he took, ordered ice to be brought, and told [Ibn al-Aghlab] to fill himself up with it; then he made him vomit, and all the milk which had turned into cheese through the coldness of the ice came out. Isḥāq said: "O Emir! Had that milk entered the tubes of your lungs and stuck there, you would have died of suffocation; but I congealed it and extracted it before it got that far". Ziyādatallāh [Ibn al-Aghlab], however, said: "Isḥāq has auctioned my soul—stop paying him!" When his payment was stopped, [Isḥāq] went off to a spacious place in one of the large squares of Kairouan, where he set up a chair, an inkwell and sheets of paper, and spent the

---

354 *Nuzhat al-nafs*, copied by ṢAṬab 61,2 and IAU 3.2/1000,3f.

355 Read *mālankhūliyā* (< *μελαγχολία*), instead of *mālakhūniyā*. The 'clarification' given in ŶulGen 122 note 120 ("Actualmente esta enfermedad se conoce con el nombre de Neurastenia") is misleading.

356 This is a reference to Isḥāq's famous and highly influential *Maqāla fī l-Mālankhūliyā* "Treatise on Melancholia" (see UllMed 125 and GaS 3/266 no. 1), conceived as an enhancement of Rufus of Ephesus' (fl. around 100 CE) *Περὶ μελαγχολίας* and, in that sense, not actually 'unprecedented' (*lam yusbaq ilā mithlihī*).

357 *Fī l-Faṣd*, see GaS 3/267 no. 6.

358 *Fī l-Nabḍ*, see GaS 3/267 no. 7.

359 In the Maghreb, one *mithqāl* equalled 4.7 g of gold, slightly more than the 'canonical' weight of the gold dinar (4.2 g), see HiMW 2 and 10.

day writing prescriptions in exchange for gold dinars. [When] somebody said to Ziyādatallāh [Ibn al-Aghlab]: "You have made Isḥāq rich", he had him arrested [and thrown] into prison, but the people followed him there. At nighttime, then, [Ibn al-Aghlab] had him taken out [and brought] before himself.

[It was then that] they argued and blamed each other, until Ziyādatallāh [Ibn al-Aghlab] got so angry with [Isḥāq] that he ordered to bleed ﴿٨٦﴾ both his forearms—and so he bled to death; [then Ibn al-Aghlab] ordered his [corpse] to be crucified on the same beams of wood on which al-Fazārī had been crucified.[360]

Abū Jaʿfar Aḥmad ibn Ibrāhīm [Ibn al-Jazzār][361] said: "Isḥāq remained on the cross for such a long time that a falcon made its nest in his belly". [Isḥāq] had a long beard whose hair did not fall out, and which swayed in the wind. Among the things he said to Ziyādatallāh [Ibn al-Aghlab] that night was: "O Gloomster![362] By God, you claim to be the chief of the Arabs, but you are no chief for them!"; and: "For ages I fed you a drug to mess up your mind!" Ziyādatallāh [Ibn al-Aghlab], who was [already] mad, fell into melancholia[363] and died [soon after].

﴿٨٧﴾ 33
Isḥāq ibn Sulaymān the Israelite[364]

An Egyptian oculist at first, he [later] settled in Kairouan, became a devoted student of Isḥāq ibn ʿImrān,[365] and [also] rendered medical services to ʿUbaydallāh the Shīʿite.[366] [Isḥāq] was an eloquent physician; he knew about the

360 Ibrāhīm al-Fazārī (not to be confused with the famous 2nd/8th century astronomer) was a 'freethinking', mocking poet from Kairouan; he was at some point accused of apostacy and sentenced to crucifixion by a judge who died in the year 275/888: al-Fazārī's throat was slit, he was bound upside down to a cross, and finally cremated (!), see ʿIyTM 4/313,11–22.

361 See biography **34** below.

362 *malkhūnī* is a somewhat irregular derivation of the neologistic root ∗(*ta*)*malkhana*∗ "to suffer from / be seized by melancholia".

363 *tamalkhana*, cf. the preceding note.

364 Abū Yaʿqūb Isḥāq ibn Sulaymān 'the Israelite', a physician and Neoplatonic philosopher, was born around the year 241/855 in Egypt; he emigrated to Kairouan at about the age of fifty, and died there around the year 344/955 (not "aproximadamente el 320/932" [ŶulGen 122 note 122]), see UllMed 137 f., GaS 3/295 ff. and AltIS *passim*.

365 See biography **32** above.

366 That is the founder and first caliph of the Fāṭimid dynasty in North Africa, Abū Muḥammad ʿUbaydallāh (or ʿAbdallāh) ibn al-Ḥusayn al-Mahdī bi-llāh (reg. 296/909–322/934); note that Sunnite authors like Ibn Juljul often use the diminutive (and pejorative) form *ʿUbaydallāh* (instead of *ʿAbdallāh*).

divisions of speech and the derivation of meanings. He lived over one hundred years. He never took a wife, nor fathered a child. He [authored several] writings, the likes of some of which nobody had [produced] before, such as: his book [titled] *On Urine*, the most satisfactory work [on this subject] any author had ever written—with it, he surpassed all [his] predecessors;[367] or his book *On Fevers*;[368] or his book *On Food and Drug*[*s*].[369] He [also wrote] philosophical works, among them: his book which he called *The Garden of Wisdom*;[370] or his book [titled] *On Definitions*;[371] or his book *On Logic*;[372] or his book *On the Theriac*.[373]

[When] he was asked: "Would you not be happy if you had a child?", he said: "Now that I have accomplished the *Book on Fevers*,[374] [I need] nothing more"—by which he meant that the perpetuation of his memory was better served by the *Book on Fevers* than by a child.

﴾٨٨﴿ 34
Abū Jaʿfar

Aḥmad ibn Ibrāhīm ibn Abī Khālid al-Jazzār[375] [was] a resident of Kairouan, a Muslim by faith, a physician, the son of a physician, and his uncle Abū Bakr [also practised medicine].[376] He was one of those who met Isḥāq ibn Sulay-

367 *Fī l-Bawl*, see UllMed 138 and GaS 3/296 f. no. 3.

368 *Fī l-Ḥummayāt*, Isḥāq's masterpiece, see UllMed 137 f. and Gas 3/296 no. 1.

369 *Fī l-Ghidhāʾ wa-l-dawāʾ*, most probably identical with the *Kitāb al-Aghdhiya* "Book on Foodstuffs", see UllMed 200 and GaS 3/296 no. 2; cf. IAU 3.2/1002,-3 f. with 1005 no. 2: *Kitāb al-Adwiya wa-l-aghdhiya* "Book on Drugs and Foodstuffs".

370 *Bustān al-ḥikma*, apparently a metaphysical work, see ṢATab 88,13 f. and IAU 3.2/1005 no. 7.

371 *Fī l-Ḥudūd*, full title … *wa-l-rusūm* "and descriptions", see AltIS *passim* with ṢATab 88,13 and IAU 3.2/1005 no. 6.

372 *Fī l-Manṭiq*, cf. IAU 3.2/1005 no. 8: *al-Tadakhkhul ilā l-manṭiq* "Introduction to Logic".

373 *Fī l-Tiryāq*, cf. IAU 3.2/1005 no. 11.

374 Cf. note 368 above.

375 Generally known as *Ibn al-Jazzār* (ṢATab 61,17); he died in the year 369/979, aged eighty-something, see UllMed 147 ff., GaS 3/304–307 and IdIDj *passim*. Note that the date given for Ibn al-Jazzār's death by Ullmann and Idris (opp.cit.), namely 395/1004, cannot be right: Ibn Juljul completed his *Generations* in the year 377/987 and yet, at the end of the present biographical entry, he was able to record Ibn al-Jazzār's age *when he died* (Sezgin [op.cit.] already made this point, but it is worth repeating).

376 Nothing is known about Ibn al-Jazzār's father; as for his uncle, Abū Bakr Muḥammad ibn Abī Khālid, he left a few compound prescriptions (potions, electuaries, theriacs) which the nephew incorporated into an otherwise unattested (but preserved) work called "Medicine for Old Men" (*Ṭibb al-mashāyikh*), see JulṬab 90 note 1 = UllMed 148 and GaS 3/306 no. 7 (full title … *wa-ḥifẓ ṣiḥḥatihim* "and the preservation of their health").

mān[377] and associated with him. On medicine, he [wrote several] ﴾٨٩﴿ wonderful works.[378] He was endowed with a good memory, an inquisitive mind, keen to learn medicine as well as other sciences—[thus] he [also wrote some] works on non-medical [topics], such as his chronicles[379] and his book [titled] *Aphorisms and Elegant Sayings*.[380]

[Ibn al-Jazzār] adopted for himself an admirable attitude with regard to his appearance, his conduct, and his restraint. Not once was he ensnared by temptation whilst in Kairouan, nor did he indulge in pleasures. He attended funerals and weddings, but never ate [anything] there. He would not travel to [see] any men in North Africa, not [even] a ruler, with the exception of Abū Ṭālib, the uncle of Maʿadd,[381] who was an old friend of his and whom he visited on Fridays, but only then. Every year he embarked on a journey to Monastir, [to] a fortified place of retreat by the sea,[382] where he stayed for the duration of midsummer; then he returned to Kairouan.[383] Over the door of his house he fixed a rooflet, under which he installed one of his servants, [a man] who went by the name of Rashīq, and who prepared in his presence all electuaries, potions and [other such compound] drugs. In the morning, [Ibn al-Jazzār] would examine [urine] flasks, [then] tell [his patients] to pass by the servant and receive from him [their] medicine; in doing so, he made sure that he personally did not take any [payment] from anyone.[384]

[The following story] I was told by somebody I trust. He said: "One morning, I was in [Ibn al-Jazzār's] reception room, which was crammed with people,

---

377 See biography **33** above.

378 For these see UllMed 147ff. and GaS 3/304–307 (30 titles).

379 This seems to be a collective reference to Ibn al-Jazzār's *Akhbār al-dawla* (a history of the Fāṭimid dynasty), *Maghāzī Ifrīqiya* (on the Arab conquest of North Africa) and *al-Taʿrīf bi-ṣaḥīḥ al-taʾrīkh* (containing obituaries and historical anecdotes), see IAU 3.2/1008f. nos 6 and 26 with IdIDj *passim*.

380 *al-Fuṣūl wa-l-balāghāt*, full title *al-Fuṣūl fī sāʾir al-ʿulūm wa-l-balāghāt* "Aphorisms on Various Sciences and Elegant Sayings", cf. IAU 3.2/1009 no. 27.

381 That is the fourth Fāṭimid caliph Abū Tamīm *Maʿadd* ibn Ismāʿīl al-Muʿizz li-Dīn Allāh (reg. 341/953–365/975). The reading *Muʿidd* (instead of Maʿadd)—as given in ŶulGen 83,16 and 85,5—is to be emended.

382 This is a reference to the famous *Ribat of Monastir*, founded in 796 CE by the ʿAbbāsid general Harthama ibn Aʿyan.

383 The text here reads *Ifrīqiya* "central North Africa", but the context requires the emendation *al-Qayrawān* "Kairouan".

384 It is not clear whether this statement indicates that Ibn al-Jazzār, in his capacity as a general practitioner, refused to be paid *on principle*, or whether he refused to be paid *directly*.

when the nephew of the judge al-Nuʿmān[385] walked in—this was an important young man in North Africa, whom the judge had nominated as his replacement in case something prevented him from the administration of justice. There was no other place for him to sit in the reception than the seat of Abū Jaʿfar [Ibn al-Jazzār]. When the latter came out [of his office] and the nephew of the judge rose to his feet, he was not invited to remain seated or to make himself comfortable. He showed [Ibn al-Jazzār] a flask he had [brought] with him, containing the urine of his cousin, al-Nuʿmān's son, and received a detailed answer about it, all the while standing. Then he mounted [his animal] and took off. He bore no grudge [towards Ibn al-Jazzār] over this matter, [in fact] he kept coming back every day with [his cousin's] urine, until the patient was cured".

My informant [further] said: "I was in the company [of Ibn al-Jazzār] one midmorning when a messenger from the judge al-Nuʿmān entered with a letter in which he thanked him for having taken care of the treatment of his son; [the messenger] also brought a bundle containing a robe and three hundred *mithqāl*.[386] [Ibn al-Jazzār] read the letter and replied gratefully, but he accepted neither the money nor the robe".

My informant went on: "[When] I told him: 'Abū Jaʿfar! This is a godsend blessing and you reject it?', he said to me: 'By God, no man from Maʿadd's[387] clan shall do me a favour!'" [Ibn al-Jazzār] lived more than eighty ﴿٩٠﴾ years. After his death, they found that he possessed twenty-four thousand gold dinars and twenty-five *qinṭār*[388] of medical books and others. He had planned to emigrate to al-Andalus but could not make it happen. He lived during the reign of Maʿadd.[389]

﴿٩٢﴾ The **ninth generation**: sages and physicians of al-Andalus

Medicine in al-Andalus used to rely on a book of the Christians that was [later] translated [into Arabic], and that bore the title *Aphorisms*, meaning 'collection'

385 al-Nuʿmān ibn Muḥammad al-Tamīmī (d. 363/974), also known as Ibn Ḥayyūn, was the powerful judge (later judge-in-chief [*qāḍī l-quḍāh*]) of the Fāṭimid caliph al-Muʿizz li-Dīn Allāh, see DaNuʿ *passim*; on al-Muʿizz cf. note 381 above.

386 On *mithqāl* see note 359 above.

387 Cf. note 381 above.

388 In the Maghreb, under the Fāṭimids, one *qinṭār* equalled 43.7 kg, see HiMW 39 and 47; accordingly, 25 *qinṭār* add up to 1092 kg.

389 Cf. note 381 above.

or 'compilation'.[390] In the days of ʿAbd al-Raḥmān ibn al-Ḥakam,[391] some Christians practised medicine, but they had no deeper insight into its sophisticated form, nor [did they understand] philosophy and geometry.

[Then], in the days of the emir Muḥammad,[392] medicine was cultivated by

﴾٩٣﴿ 35
Ḥamdīn ibn Ubbā[393]

He was a skilled, experienced physician, related by marriage to the Banū Khālid.[394] He had estates and revenues in Córdoba. He never rode an animal unless it had been bred in his [stables], never ate anything unless it had been [grown] on his soil, never wore anything unless it had been [woven] from the linen of his land, and never took into service anyone other than the houseborn sons of his slaves.

---

390 (*al-*)*Aburīshim* is probably a transliteration of *Ἀφορισμοί*, scil. Hippocrates' selfsame work which was translated into Arabic, in the Islamic East, around the middle of the 3rd/9th century by Ḥunayn ibn Isḥāq under the title *al-Fuṣūl* lit. "Divisions", cf. FiCH 21ff. no. 13. Ibn Juljul's transliteration seems to suggest that this work, in the Islamic West, circulated under a different title, which was moreover influenced by Old Castilian (consider the transition from *s* to *sh*); and the given explanation of *Aburīshim*, viz. "collection (*majmūʿ*) or compilation (*jāmiʿ*)", indicates that Ibn Juljul must have had only a dim notion of the term's original meaning, and only a vague idea of the work's structure and contents. Note in passing the interesting proposition made JanNMD 1/124, namely that ابريشم may be a corruption of a Latin intermediate form representing the title *Euporista* (i.q. *Περὶ εὐπορίστων*), a work on commonly used drugs by Oribasius (d. 403 CE)—which would obviously imply the availability of a Latin translation of that text in Muslim Spain by the middle of the 3rd/9th century, at the latest. However, since the term (*al-*)*Aburīshim* reoccurs in biography **43** as the title of a medical writing by the Andalusian physician Yaḥyā ibn Isḥāq (fl. early 4th/10th century), an *aphoristic* connotation seems much more likely.

391 That is the fourth Umayyad emir of Córdoba, ʿAbd al-Raḥmān II ibn al-Ḥakam (reg. 206/822–238/852).

392 That is the fifth Umayyad emir of Córdoba, Muḥammad I ibn ʿAbd al-Raḥmān (reg. 238/852–273/886).

393 Ḥamdīn ibn Ubbā (VerMA 454 note 74: "Ubbâ = Oppas"?) is primarily known through Ibn Juljul's present account, which Ibn Abī Uṣaybiʿa, among others, copied almost literally, see IAU 3.2/1017. Ḥamdīn, being a contemporary of Muḥammad I (cf. the preceding note), flourished around the middle of the 3rd/9th century.

394 The Banū Khālid were a prestigious family of Umayyad 'clients' who wielded considerable power throughout the emirates and caliphates of Córdoba; their history has been traced in magnificent detail by PuerLP 61–129 (Ḥamdīn ibn Ubbā figures there, implicitly after Ibn Juljul, as a physician "de probable origen mozárabe, que era yerno de los Banū Jālid, aunque no sabemos de que individuo en concreto" [op.cit. 129 no. 40 with note 197]).

36
Jawād the Christian physician[395]

He lived in the days of the emir Muḥammad.[396] There is a linctus[397] attributed to Jawād; his is [moreover the so-called] *monk's remedy*;[398] and [there are several] potions[399] attributed to him and [also] to Ḥamdīn[400]—the potion of Ḥamdīn [contains] one hundred and one simple drugs, all herbal.

﴿٩٤﴾ 37
al-Ḥarrānī[401] who arrived from the East

in the days of the emir Muḥammad.[402] [al-Ḥarrānī] is the one who built the mosque that is named after him, meaning the Ḥarrānī mosque, which lies next to the Qmrī mosque,[403] and which is where his house stood. He brought to al-Andalus an electuary to [treat] abdominal pains, which he sold for fifty[404] gold dinars per dose, making good money with it. Five physicians—Ḥamdīn,[405] Jawād,[406] and [some] others—got together and collected fifty gold dinars, in

395 Jawād (fl. mid 3rd/9th century) is primarily known through Ibn Juljul's present account, which Ibn Abī Uṣaybiʿa paraphrased, see IAU 3.2/1017 f.

396 Cf. note 392 above.

397 Arabic *laʿūq*.

398 Arabic *dawāʾ al-rāhib*.

399 Arabic *bassūnāt*, pl. of *bassūn* < *poción* (?), cf. DoSupp 1/87b.

400 See biography 35 above.

401 That is Yūnus ibn Aḥmad al-Ḥarrānī (fl. late 3rd/9th century). His full name is given later on by Ibn Juljul, when he deals with Yūnus' two sons (see biography 55/56 below), and it is also recorded, in the same context, by ṢATab 80,18; QifTaʾ 394,20 ('Yūnus' only) with 395,18; and IAU 3.2/1021,1–4. Note that Ṣāʿid al-Andalusī, elsewhere in his book (ṢATab 78,11 f.), says that "a man from Ḥarrān arrived who became known in al-Andalus [simply] as 'al-Ḥarrānī'—his [personal] name has not come down to me (*lam yablughnī ʾsmuhū*)"; cf. further GaS 3/258.

402 Cf. note 392 above.

403 VerMA 454 no. 37,3 with note 84 reads *al-Qumarī*—this reading (القمري) is confirmed by the Andalusian writer Ibn Ḥazm (d. 456/1064), who says the mosque was located "on the western side" (*bi-l-jānib al-gharbī*) of Córdoba, see IḤṬawq 286,1 (Arberry: *al-Qamarī*); however, Iḥsān ʿAbbās, the editor of Ibn Ḥazm's *Ṭawq*, prefers to read the name as *al-ʿUmarī* (العمري), see loc.cit. note 2 (with the literature quoted there). The Qmrī mosque is not registered in the detailed list of Córdoban mosques given by LéPrEM 208 f. note 2. ŶulGen 123 f. note 136 is also at a loss.

404 Read *bi-khamsīna* (instead of *bi-khsyn*, a printing error).

405 See biography 35 above.

406 See biography 36 above.

order to buy a dose of this drug. Each one of them walked away with a [sample] portion, smelled it, tasted it, and [they all separately] recorded what their senses had led them to conclude about it. Later they met again, agreed on their conjectures [regarding the drug's composition], and wrote that down. Then they went to al-Ḥarrānī and said to him: "God has allowed you to benefit from this drug whose [composition] you alone know. We are physicians who bought from you ﴿٩٥﴾ a dose [of it]; we did this and that, and came to such and such a conclusion. If our conjectures are correct, then we have cracked it; if not, share with us [your] knowledge of its [composition], for you have already drawn profit [from it]".[407] [al-Ḥarrānī] asked to be shown their formula, then said: "You have not missed any of the ingredients, but you have failed to determine their right proportions. The drug is known as *great helper*".[408] He shared its composition with them, and from then on it became common in al-Andalus. I have seen [an account of] this story in the possession of Abū l-Aṣbagh al-Rāzī, handwritten by al-Mustanṣir bi-llāh, the Commander of the Faithful—may God have mercy upon him.[409]

There is another anecdote that involves him, to wit: [one day] a pharmaceutical prescription was found in which [it said] 'take such and such [an amount] of *thuffāʾ*', but nobody knew what *thuffāʾ* was. So they went to [al-Ḥarrānī] and asked him: "Do you have *thuffāʾ*?" [When] he replied "Yes", they asked: "How much costs a weight of two *dirham*[410] of it?" He said: "Ten gold dinars", and once he had taken [the money], he presented them with garden cress. They said to him: "This is garden cress! We know that!" And he replied: "I did not charge you for the drug as such, but for the explanation of its name".[411]

---

407 The phrase *fa-qad intafaʿta* "for you have already drawn profit (from it)" is found in Ibn Abī Uṣaybiʿa's parallel version (IAU 2.2/915,9) and has been inserted into Ibn Juljul's text by its editor, for good reasons.

408 Arabic *al-mughīth al-kabīr*, cf. DoSupp 2/230b; according to JulṬab 95 note 7, the drug was called 'helper' because it did to the cardinal organs what heavy rain does to parched land.

409 Abū l-Aṣbagh ʿĪsā ibn Aḥmad al-Rāzī (d. 379/989) was a historian and secretary to the second Umayyad caliph of Córdoba, al-Ḥakam II ibn ʿAbd al-Raḥmān al-Mustanṣir bi-llāh (reg. 350/961–366/976), see AbbTak 3/419 no. 2878.

410 The 'canonical' weight of the *dirham* equalled 3.125 g; in the Maghreb and in Muslim Spain, however, it was set at 3.3 g, see HiMW 4 and 10.

411 *thuffāʾ* is a (lesser known) synonym of *ḥurf* "garden cress" (*Lepidium sativum*), see SchMM 163 no. 239; according to Ibn al-Bayṭār (*apud* DoSupp 1/159b), *thuffāʾ* was the name given to that plant by the inhabitants of the Hejaz (!).

﴿٩٦﴾ 38
Khālid ibn Yazīd

ibn Rūmān the Christian.[412] He was highly skilled in medicine and one of its champions at the time. He lived [close to] the church of San Acisclo,[413] in a building that is known [today] as 'the house of the poet Ibn al-Shaṭajayrī'.[414] Thanks to medicine, he acquired wealth and estates. Next to his residence, he built a [public] bathhouse named after him. He was a dexterous maker [of drugs], and [particularly] knowledgeable about herbal substances, which brought [many] benefits to the community. Nasṭās ibn Jurayj, the Egyptian physician,[415] wrote for him an epistle [titled] *On Urine*.[416] Khālid was succeeded by a son, whom he had named Yazīd;[417] the latter [however] did not excel at medicine as much as his father.

﴿٩٧﴾ 39
Ibn Malūka the Christian[418]

His residence was known as 'the house of the postmaster Khalaf',[419] [located] by the water-worn bank of the river [Guadalquivir]. He lived during the final days of the emir 'Abdallāh[420] and at the beginning of the reign of the emir 'Abd al-Raḥmān al-Nāṣir.[421] He used to make [drugs] with his own hands,

412 For a (slightly abridged) parallel account on Khālid ibn Yazīd, a physician who lived around the middle of the 4th/10th century in Córdoba, see IAU 3.2/1018; cf. also GaS 3/303.

413 Arabic *Shant Ajlj* (اجلج < *اججلو*?). The exact location of this church is not known—it may have stood in the suburb of the Parchment Makers, or inside the walled city to the northeast of the Cathedral of Córdoba, see LéPrEM 201 and SaSiMC 8 note 34.

414 The Andalusian poet Ḥabīb ibn Aḥmad al-Shaṭajayrī, a much younger contemporary of the caliph al-Mustanṣir (cf. note 409 above), died before or around the year 430/1038, see ḤumJM 175 no. 392.

415 See biography **31** above.

416 Cf. note 348 above.

417 Not known otherwise.

418 Ibn Juljul's present account on Ibn Malūka is the oldest we possess; for a trimmed version of it see IAU 3.2/1018.

419 Not known otherwise.

420 That is the seventh Umayyad emir of Córdoba, 'Abdallāh ibn Muḥammad (reg. 275/888–300/912).

421 That is the last Umayyad emir and first caliph of Córdoba, 'Abd al-Raḥmān III ibn Muḥam-

and performed venesections. At the door of his house [were placed] thirty chairs for seating patients.

40
Isḥāq the physician[422]

[He was] the father of the vizier Ibn Isḥāq.[423] His residence was close to the mosque of Ṭāhir.[424] He was a Christian by faith. He was a dexterous maker [of drugs], and [very] experienced. Great benefactions and marvellous exploits are reported of him; [in terms of] practical skill, he surpassed all his contemporaries. [Isḥāq] lived in the days of the emir ʿAbdallāh.[425] Then came the reign of al-Nāṣir li-Dīn Allāh ﴾٩٨﴿ ʿAbd al-Raḥmān ibn Muḥammad,[426] in whose days one [divine] blessing followed the other: books on medicine and all sciences arrived from the East, aroused great interest, and famous physicians appeared [already] at the beginning of his reign.

41
ʿImrān ibn Abī ʿUmar[427]

He resided in Shblār.[428] He was a noble-minded physician who rendered medical service to the emir ʿAbd al-Raḥmān al-Nāṣir,[429] and who fabricated for

mad al-Nāṣir li-Dīn Allāh (reg. 300/912–316/929 [as emir] and 316/929–350/961 [as caliph]).

422 Isḥāq lived in Córdoba in the late 3rd/9th century—for an abridged version of Ibn Juljul's account see IAU 3.2/1022; cf. further ṢAṬab 78,15 and QifTa' 359,16 f.

423 See biography **43** below.

424 According to a remark at the beginning of biography **49**, this mosque stood in a suburb (*rabaḍ*) of Córdoba; Ibn al-Abbār mentions a Córdoban mosque called *al-Ẓāfir* "the Triumphant" (AbbTak 4/71,10), but neither of them is registered in the detailed list of mosques given by LéPrEM 208 f. note 2. Consider that Arabic طاهر and ظافر are easily confused.

425 Cf. note 420 above.

426 Cf. note 421 above.

427 ʿImrān, apparently a blind man (from birth?), was physician-cum-jester at the court in Córdoba; he died in the year 320/932, see FagBM 2/345 f. with LéPrEM 51 note 3. Ibn Juljul's present account reappears IAU 3.2/1019; cf. further GaS 3/301.

428 Shblār was an eastern suburb (*rabaḍ*) of Córdoba, see FarTa' 1/272,9 with note 1: *Shiblād*; BashṢi 2/105,2: *Shablār*; YāBul 3/322 [after Ibn al-Faraḍī]: *Shblād* "a village (*qarya*) in al-Andalus"; LéPrEM 207 note 3 no. 10: *Šubullār*; VerMA 456 no. 41,1: *Šublār*.

429 Cf. note 421 above.

him the [so-called] *aniseed* pills.[430] He was a learned, intelligent [man]. He [authored] a medical writing in the style of a compendium.[431]

﴿٩٩﴾ 42
Muḥammad ibn Fatḥ Ṭumlūn[432]

He was a client[433] of ʿImrān ibn Abī ʿUmar.[434] He excelled at medicine to such a degree that he surpassed [all] his contemporaries, though he did not serve as physician [to the court][435]—when he was asked [to enter royal service], he excused himself, appealing directly to the emir, and was in the end exempted. Not a single person of distinction in his time could forgo his assistance.

[The following story] I was told by Abū l-Aṣbagh Ibn Ḥayyawayh.[436] He said: "I found myself in the company of the vizier ʿAbdallāh ibn Badr,[437] whose son Muḥammad[438] was afflicted with ulcers that had spread all over his body. Several physicians were present, including Ṭumlūn. Each one of them gave his opinion about this ulceration and its [possible] cause, [only] Ṭumlūn remained silent. [When] the vizier asked him: 'What do you make of it? I see you say noth-

430 Note that in biography 48 below, Ibn Juljul associates the fabrication of these pills with the physician Aṣbagh ibn Yaḥyā. A pharmacopoeia from the Islamic East, written around the middle of the 3rd/9th century, specifies the preparation of a compound drug which ran under the trade name of "*aniseed* pastilles", and which was employed to treat gastric disorders, see SābDis 110 no. 196—did this famous pharmacopoeia travel together with the "books on medicine … from the East" which began to arrive in al-Andalus, according to Ibn Juljul (see biography 40 above), at the beginning of the 4th/10th century?

431 *ka-l-kunnāsh*. Note that if the word *ta'līf* is read as a plural (viz. *ta'ālīf*, Arabic تاليف for both), the sentence may be translated "He (authored) medical writings, for example the *Compendium*"—Vernet glosses over the problem, mistakes *kunnāsh* for a plural, and translates: *compuso un libro de medicina como los «cuadernos»* (VerMA 456 no. 41,4).

432 Ṭumlūn (VerMA 456 no. 42,1: Ṭamlūn) was a physician in Córdoba who lived at the beginning of the 4th/10th century. Ibn Juljul's present account was copied verbatim by IAU 3.2/1019; the latter, in turn, served as a source for al-Ṣafadī's brief entry on Ṭumlūn, cf. ṢafWā 4/224 no. 1864.

433 On the term *mawlan* "client" cf. note 263 above.

434 See biography 41 above.

435 VerMA 456 no. 42,3 misleadingly translates this phrase by "pero no ejercía"; similarly ŶulGen 90,-9.

436 He is almost certainly identical with the Andalusian scholar Abū l-Aṣbagh ʿĪsā ibn Muḥammad Ibn Ḥayyawayh (d. 374/985), a contemporary of Ibn Juljul, see FarTa' 1/431 f. no. 987. In the text, read *Ḥayyawayh* (instead of *Khywy* [خيوى]); in ŶulGen 90,-5 emend the reading *Jayaway*.

437 Is he the same as ʿAbdallāh ibn Badr, chief of the police in Córdoba until he was sacked by the caliph al-Ḥakam II (FagBM 2/388 with LéPrEM 105 f.)?

438 Not known otherwise.

ing!', he replied: 'I have an ointment[439] which will heal these ulcers without delay'. [The vizier], who inclined to [heed] his advice, ordered him to bring the ointment and to apply it to the ulcers, which [indeed] dried up that very night. And so ʿAbdallāh ibn Badr awarded him fifty gold dinars and clad him in a robe [of honour], whereas the other physicians walked away empty-handed".

﴿١٠٠﴾ 43
Yaḥyā ibn Isḥāq[440]

He was a noble-minded, knowledgeable, manually skilled physician. He lived at the beginning of the reign of al-Nāṣir,[441] who appointed him vizier. [Yaḥyā also] was in charge of [certain] provinces and [tax] districts, and for a while he was military chief of Badajoz. The Commander of the Faithful, al-Nāṣir, held him in high esteem, granted him a position of trust, and allowed him to look after [his] wives and concubines.

A reliable source told me that he had a servant [who used to work] for the chamberlain Mūsā[442] or for the vizier ʿAbd al-Malik,[443] [and that this servant] had said: "[One day] my master sent me to [Yaḥyā ibn Isḥāq] with a letter. I was sitting at the door of his house, by the Walnut Gate,[444] when a screaming peasant on a donkey approached, came ever closer, finally stopped at the door of the house, and started to beg [for my help], saying: 'Please listen to me! [Go] inform the vizier of my condition!' Alerted by the man's cries, [Yaḥyā] came out, car-

439 Vernet, having correctly translated *marham* by "pomada" (VerMA 456 no. 42,10), proceeds to embark on a rather futile speculation (loc.cit. note 103), namely that this term may be identical with (a corrupt hapax) *marhamar*, which occurs in al-Kindī's (d. ca. 256/870) dispensatory (KinAq 48 no. 23 with 336 no. 288) as an ingredient of a compound ointment (*ṭaly*) to treat erysipelas (*ḥumra*). al-Kindī's term, by the way, is likely to reflect a clerical error for *murr murr* "bitter myrrh", or else a dittography of *murr*.

440 Yaḥyā, the son of 'Isḥāq the physician' (see biography 40 above), was also a high-ranking government functionary, administrator and commissioned officer who lived in the early decades of the 4th/10th century; unlike his father, who was a Christian, Yaḥyā became a Muslim. Ibn Juljul's account on him is the oldest and best we possess, but still see ṢAṬab 78,14–17; QifTa' 359 f.; IAU 3.2/1023 ff.; and, for some further sources, VerMA 456 note 104.

441 al-Nāṣir's reign as emir began in the year 300/912, his reign as caliph began in the year 316/929; cf. note 421 above.

442 Mūsā ibn Muḥammad Ibn Ḥudayr, chamberlain and since 300/912 vizier of ʿAbd al-Raḥmān III al-Nāṣir, died in the year 320/932, see FagBM 2/263, 302, 345 and *passim* with LéPrEM 101.

443 ʿAbd al-Malik ibn Jahwar was appointed vizier by ʿAbd al-Raḥmān III al-Nāṣir in the year 305/918, see FagBM 2/284 with LéPrEM 100 note 2.

444 The Walnut Gate (*Bāb al-Jawz*) was one of the seven gates in the city wall of Córdoba and also known as 'Badajoz Gate', see GayHis 1/369 and LéPrEM 204 f.; further BashṢi 2/125,6.

rying [his] reply to the letter I [had delivered]. He asked the man: 'What is the matter with you, eh?' 'O Vizier!', replied [the man], 'A swelling in my penis[445] shackles me, I have not been able to urinate for many days now, and I am on the brink of death!' [Yaḥyā] said: 'Show me!' And the man uncovered his penis, which was swollen indeed. Then [Yaḥyā turned] to the person who was accompanying the patient [and] said: 'Find me a smooth stone!' Having searched [and found] one, he brought it to the vizier, who said: 'Hold [that stone] in the palm of your hand and put [the patient's] penis on top of it!'" [My source went on to] say that his [own] source continued [as follows]: "Once the man's penis was firmly placed on the stone, the vizier made a fist and hit the penis with such force that the patient lost consciousness. Pus began to flow,[446] and immediately thereafter urine.[447] [When] the man opened his eyes [again], [Yaḥyā] said to him: 'Go now, you are cured of your affliction, but never come back—you are a wicked man, you sodomized a beast ﴿١٠١﴾ and by chance encountered a grain from its fodder, which got stuck inside [your] penis and caused it to swell; [the grain] has come out with the pus'. The man replied: 'Ah, yes! That's how it was and that's what I did', and he admitted his [misdoings]". This [story] indicates the soundness of [Yaḥyā's] intuition, and the purity, finesse, eminence and brilliance of [his] talent.

[Yaḥyā] wrote a medical compendium in five volumes, following the [didactic] method of the Byzantines, [and] calling it *Aphorisms*.[448] [There is another] cherished anecdote about him, involving the treatment of al-Nāṣir[449]—may God be pleased with him:

[Once] al-Nāṣir suffered from an earache—[this happened] at a time when the vizier [Yaḥyā] was still military chief of Badajoz. al-Nāṣir received treatment, but [as the pain] did not subside, he ordered to send for [Yaḥyā]. The messenger[450] departed, and [upon his arrival] said to [Yaḥyā]: "Quick, get ready!" [When the latter] very politely asked for the reason he was being called,

445 Strictly speaking, the term *iḥlīl* denotes the urethra, but in the context of this story (and some others) it is clearly used as a euphemism (or colloquialism?) for "penis".

446 The editor of Ibn Juljul's text here inserted the unnecessary phrase *fa-mā 'stawfā l-rajul jary^{a} ṣadīd al-waram ḥattā fataḥa 'aynayhī* "the man was not aware of the flowing of pus from the swelling until he opened his eyes (again)", obtained from IAU 2.2/918,6 (cf. JulṬab 102 note 17); VerMA 457 note 108 also recognized this phrase to be redundant but strangely translates it "y el hombre volvió en sí cuando aún salía el pus (…)".

447 Read *thumma l-bawl* (instead of *thumma bāla l-bawl*).

448 *(al-)Aburīshim* < Ἀφορισμοί, cf. also note 390 above.

449 Cf. note 421 above.

450 *furāniq* "messenger" is a somewhat unusual arabicized Persian term, viz. *parwānak* "a messenger, courier, running footman", see StDic 245a–b.

the messenger replied: "The Commander of the Faithful suffers from an earache that defies the physicians!" On his way [to Córdoba], [Yaḥyā] made a detour [and visited] one of the Christian monasteries, where he enquired about a [certain] savant. He met with a man of advanced age whom he asked: "Do you have any experience in treating earache?" The old monk replied: "[Use] warm pigeon blood!" Then [Yaḥyā] joined the Commander of the Faithful, treated him with the warm, flowing blood of a [freshly slaughtered] pigeon, and [the patient] was cured.

If you look at this [story], you will find that it [speaks] of admirable investigation, utmost diligence, and tireless devotion to learning.[451]

﴿١٠٢﴾ 44
Abū Bakr Sulaymān Ibn Bāj[452]

He lived during the reign of al-Nāṣir[453]—may God have mercy upon him—and rendered medical service to this [ruler]. He was a noble-minded physician. He treated al-Nāṣir, the Commander of the Faithful—may God be pleased with him—for a nasty eye inflammation with a collyrium [that cured him] in a day; later he was asked [to share] the formula [of this drug], but he refused to dictate it. He treated the postmaster Shunayf[454] for shortness of breath with a linctus [that cured him] in a day, after [other physicians] had failed to do so. He used to treat hip pain with a pill [that cured it] in good time.[455] Yet he jealously guarded [his] drug formulas. Many anecdotes about him, involving medicine, are cherished by ﴿١٠٣﴾ the community. He was a man of culture. Towards the end of his days, he amputated his penis[456] because of an [incurable] ulcer that had developed on it. The Commander of the Faithful, al-Nāṣir, entrusted him with the administration of justice in Sidonia.

---

451 Read with JulṬab 102 note 29: *al-taʿlīm* (instead of *al-takallum*, which VerMA 457 no. 43,-1 translates as "raciocinio"!).

452 Sulaymān ibn ʿAbd al-Malik ibn Bāj, physician in Córdoba and sometime judge in Sidonia, Algeciras and Ceuta, see AbbTak 4/45 no. 3114; Ibn Juljul's present account resurfaces, almost literally (and implicitly), in IAU 3.2/1025 (where the reading *Tāj* is a mistake for *Bāj* [undotted Arabic باج for both]).

453 Cf. note 421 above.

454 Perhaps identical with a former 'hospitality supervisor' (*ṣāḥib al-qirā*) from Córdoba, also named Shunayf ("Little Earring"), who was active in this particular role at the end of the 3rd/9th century and who may later have become postmaster as well, see JulṬab 103 note 2 = AbbTak 4/110 no. 3273.

455 Instead of *bi-ḥabb min ḥīnihī*, IAU 2.2/919,5 reads *bi-ḥabb min ḥabbihī* "with one of his pills"; VerMA 457 no. 44,7 f. interprets *ḥīnihī* (حينه) as *ḥīna* (حينة), translates the phrase by "con granos de *ḥīna*", but does not say what this term is supposed to denote.

456 On *iḥlīl* "penis" cf. note 445 above.

45
Ibn Umm al-Banīn[457]

We only called him 'Swellhead'.[458] He was a native of the city of Córdoba. He put the art of medicine into the service of al-Nāṣir, the Commander of the Faithful,[459] and he was his boon companion [too]. He practised medicine with intelligence—there are [many] anecdotes about him which testify[460] to that; yet he was [also] a frivolous, self-important [man]. This is why al-Nāṣir sometimes found him annoying, though at other times he clearly needed him, because of his superior intelligence. [Ibn Umm al-Banīn] was attracted to boys. An amusing story is told about him, [set against the background] of one of the military campaigns [led] by the Commander of the Faithful: ﴿١٠٤﴾ One midday, [when] he was in his tent, he approached a [young] servant of his and mounted him—lo and behold, a violent gust of wind uprooted the tents, including his own, which fell over, leaving him exposed to the people while still on top of the boy.

46
Saʿīd Ibn ʿAbd Rabbihī[461] the nephew of Aḥmad Ibn ʿAbd Rabbihī[462]

He was a noble-minded physician, a poet [and] a man of culture. On medicine, he [wrote] an excellent [poem in] *rajaz* [metre], in which he demonstrates

---

457 The editor of Ibn Juljul's text raises the possibility that Ibn Umm al-Banīn, otherwise only known through Ibn Abī Uṣaybiʿa's curtailed retelling (IAU 3.2/1025 f.), may have been a late descendant (*ibn*) of Umm al-Banīn bint ʿAbd al-ʿAzīz ibn Marwān, a wife of the sixth ruler of the (eastern) Umayyad caliphate, al-Walīd I ibn ʿAbd al-Malik (reg. 86/705–96/715), see JulṬab 103 ad 45 (citing MaqqNṬ 1.1/176,20; 181,10; and 2.1/4,14). Cf. further ṬabTa' 219,9 f. and 221,-4 f. Note in passing that *umm al-banīn* (lit. "mother of sons") is also a generic name, denoting a free-born woman, wife and mother, in contrast to *umm al-walad* (lit. "mother of a child") which denotes a slave concubine mother, see SchUW *passim*.

458 For this (and some other) connotations of the term *aʿraf* cf. LaLex 2016b–c.

459 Cf. note 421 above.

460 Read *andhara* (instead of *andara*).

461 Abū ʿUthmān Saʿīd ibn ʿAbd al-Raḥmān ibn Muḥammad ibn ʿAbd Rabbihī, a physician, astronomer and poet, was active in the first half of the 4th/10th century; he is the author of a pharmacopoeia titled *al-Dukkān* "The Drugstore" or *al-Aqrābādhīn* "The Dispensatory" (preserved), a medical poem titled *Urjūza fī l-ṭibb* (edited), and a (lost) work containing clinical notes and empirical drugs (*taʿālīq wa-mujarrabāt*); he died either in the year 342/953 or in 356/967, see UllMed 303, GaS 3/300 f. ("died ca. 350/961") and SánRa *passim*.

462 That is Abū ʿUmar Aḥmad ibn Muḥammad ibn ʿAbd Rabbihī, a famous poet, man of letters and pioneer of Arabic literature in Muslim Spain, best known for his encyclopedic work

his mastery of that science and his acquaintance with the doctrine[s] of the ancients. His method of treating fevers was to mix a bit of white chalk[463] into cooling medicines, and an elegant method it is indeed! He never served any ruler as physician. He understood prognosis, atmospheric changes, wind directions, and planetary pathways.

Sulaymān ibn Ayyūb the jurisprudent[464] told me [the following story] about him. He said: "[Once] I fell ill with a fever which affected me for a long time and had me on the brink [of death]. It so happened that [Saʿīd] passed by[465] my father on his way to [meet] the city magistrate Aḥmad ibn ʿĪsā.[466] My father went up to him, made the required salutations, and then asked him about my illness. [Saʿīd] wanted to know what treatment I was receiving. [When] my father told him, he declared my medication ridiculous, and [later] sent him eighteen pills, the ball-shaped kind, with the instruction for me to swallow a few of them every day. Yet even before I had taken the lot, my fever sailed off and I was completely cured".

﴿١٠٥﴾ One day, [Saʿīd] had to undergo venesection. He sent [a note] to his uncle Aḥmad,[467] [requesting] his company, but [the latter] did not respond and left him waiting. So [Saʿīd] composed [the following lines]:

As I lacked a friend and fellow,
I chose Hippocrates and Galen as my boon companions

And turned their books into a means to cheer me up,
because they soothe any wound that needs healing.

---

titled *al-ʿIqd* "The Necklace"; he was born in Córdoba in the year 246/860 and died there in 328/940, see HámRa *passim*.

463 *ḥawār* "white chalk" is a perfectly legitimate reading (cf. DoSupp 1/334b "craie blanche"), and Vernet's doubts about it are unfounded (VerMA 458 no. 46,5 with note 115).

464 Sulaymān ibn Ayyūb was one of Ibn Juljul's teachers in Córdoba; he died in the year 377/987, see FarTa' 1/259 f. no. 564.

465 Read *jāza* (instead of *jāra*).

466 Aḥmad ibn ʿĪsā ibn Abī ʿAbda was appointed by al-Nāṣir (cf. note 421 above) to the office of city magistrate in the year 316/928, see FagBM 2/323,-4 f. and *passim*; on the Banū Abī ʿAbda see LéPrEM 100 f. The term *ṣāḥib al-madīna*, here tentatively translated "city magistrate" (FagBM loc.cit. "préfet de la ville"), denotes an important though somewhat elusive administrative function peculiar to medieval Muslim Spain—for a detailed discussion see MeGuṢM *passim*.

467 Cf. note 462 above. After the name "Aḥmad", the editor of Ibn Juljul's text adds the dispensable specification *ibn Muḥammad ibn ʿAbd Rabbihī al-shāʿir al-adīb* "… the learned poet", which he obtained from IAU 2.2/921,10.

And I found that their knowledge, once I grasped it,
ignites and invigorates souls in their bodies.[468]

He dispatched these verses to his uncle Aḥmad who [in turn] replied with some others, of which I can only remember three. In them he says:

You found that Hippocrates and Galen
do not eat nor burden a host with expenses.

So you took them, rather than your relatives, as a protection
and were happy to let them be comrades and confidants.

I reckon your stinginess will never be seen to leave you,
such that, after their's, you sit in the company of the Devil.

al-ʿĀyidī[469]—may God have mercy upon him—recited to me [some verses], saying: [Aḥmad] Ibn ʿAbd Rabbihī recited to me [these verses] by his nephew Abū ʿUthmān [Saʿīd]:

Should I, after having delved in the sciences of truth
and longly revelled in the gifts of my Creator,

At a time when I am about to enter His kingdom,
be seen as seeking sustenance from anyone but my Sustainer?[470]

The days of a man's life are but the enjoyment of an hour
that quickly passes like a flash of lightning.[471]

My soul already announced the collapse of its saddle,
and my driver harshly urges me towards death.

---

468 The third and last verse has been added by the editor of Ibn Juljul's text from the parallel transmission of Ibn Abī Uṣaybiʿa, cf. IAU 2.2/921.

469 Yaḥyā ibn Mālik ibn ʿĀyid, known as *al-ʿĀyidī*, a native of Tortosa and highly respected traditionist, spent more than two decades travelling in the Islamic East; he returned to Spain in 369/979 and settled down in Córdoba, where he died six years later, see FarTaʾ 2/241f. no. 1598 (ibn *ʿĀʾidh*).

470 Read رازقى (instead of رازق).

471 This third verse has been inserted by the editor of Ibn Juljul's text from the parallel transmissions of Ṣāʿid al-Andalusī and Ibn Abī Uṣaybiʿa, cf. ṢAṬab 79 and IAU 2.2/922.

Even if I stood still, or swerved in flight
from death to the horizons, it would get me in the end.

[Saʿīd] was a leading figure in his profession. He became blind in his final days.

﴿١٠٧﴾ 47
Abū Ḥafṣ ʿUmar ibn Burayq[472]

He was a noble-minded physician [and] a melodious reciter of the *Koran*. He undertook a journey to Kairouan to [study under] Abū Jaʿfar Ibn al-Jazzār,[473] but he stayed with him for only six months; it was he who brought to al-Andalus the book [titled] *Provisions for the Traveller*.[474] He was highly respected in al-Andalus and rendered medical service to al-Nāṣir[475]—may God have mercy upon him. Najm ibn Ṭarafa the head falconer,[476] who had wanted [Abū Ḥafṣ] all for himself, supported him, made him rich, and introduced him into his world.

[The following piece of information] I was given by Abū Muḥammad Ibn al-Aʿmā.[477] He said: "In the morning, when Abū Ḥafṣ ibn Burayq was sitting at the door of his house to offer legal advice, I saw by his side sixteen boys, all of them Slavs.[478] He did not live long".

472 Otherwise only known through Ibn Abī Uṣaybiʿa, who copied the first paragraph of Ibn Juljul's present account almost literally, but gives the name as *ʿUmar ibn Ḥafṣ ibn Burayq*, which latter element the translators of Ibn Abī Uṣaybiʿa's work read *Barīq* (IAU 3.2/1029); Ibn al-Faraḍī registers a certain *Maḥbūb ibn Bayrīq* (*sic*, FarTaʾ 2/155 no. 1408); and Ṣāʿid al-Andalusī fleetingly mentions, in the right chronological frame, one *ʿUmar ibn Bryq* (ṢAṬab 79,-1).

473 See biography 34 above.

474 That is Ibn al-Jazzār's famous treatise *Zād al-musāfir wa-qūt al-ḥāḍir* "Provisions for the Traveller and Nourishment for the Sedentary", which was subsequently translated into Latin, Middle Greek and Hebrew, see UllMed 147 f. and GaS 3/305 f. no. 2.

475 Cf. note 421 above.

476 Not known otherwise.

477 Not known otherwise, but possibly identical with the scholar Aḥmad ibn Yaḥyā *Ibn al-Aʿmā*, who has a brief entry in FarTaʾ 1/74 no. 98 (no dates given).

478 The term *ṣaqāliba* "Slavs" may also denote, in Muslim Spain, "white eunuchs/slaves" (as opposed to *ʿabīd* "black slaves"), see MeGuṢa³ *passim*.

﴿١٠٨﴾ 48
Aṣbagh ibn Yaḥyā the physician[479]

He was a leading figure in the field of medicine, which he put into the service of al-Nāṣir[480]—may God have mercy upon him. He fabricated for al-Nāṣir, the Commander of the Faithful, the [so-called] *aniseed* pills, which have already been mentioned [as the invention] of somebody else.[481] [Aṣbagh] was a handsome, elegant old man. His testimony was accepted by the Council of Elders.[482] He was a man of integrity and honour, highly esteemed by the leaders. His residence was close to the mosque of Ṭāhir.[483]

49
Muḥammad ibn Tamlīkh[484]

He belonged to the residents of the suburb [around] the mosque of Ṭāhir.[485] He put the art of medicine into the service of al-Nāṣir.[486] He was [widely] renowned for his grasp of [prose] literature as well as metrics. The military commander Aḥmad ibn Ilyās[487] was the one who promoted him into a position of leadership.[488] [Muḥammad ibn Tamlīkh] was an elegant, calm [and]

479 Aṣbagh ibn Yaḥyā is only known through Ibn Juljul's present account, which was copied selectively, though almost literally, by Ibn Abī Uṣaybiʿa (IAU 3.2/1030) and Ibn al-Abbār (AbbTak 1/335 f. no. 548); Ṣāʿid al-Andalusī mentions only his name (ṢAṬab 79,-1 [where to read *Aṣbagh* instead of *Aṣnaʿ*, presumably a printing error]).

480 Cf. note 421 above.

481 In biography **41**, the *aniseed* pills are associated with the physician ʿImrān ibn Abī ʿUmar.

482 The phrase *fī quʿdud al-ʿudūl* "by the Council of Elders" (VerMA 460 no. 48,1 "en las asambleas de adules") has been translated IAU 3.2/1030,5 "as one of the court-assigned notary-witnesses", which seems excessive.

483 Cf. note 424 above.

484 Abū ʿAbdallāh Muḥammad ibn Tamlīkh (or *Tamlīḥ*) al-Tamīmī, a physician, grammarian, poet and traditionist from Córdoba who died in the year 361/972, see FarTaʾ 2/96 no. 1299; ṢAṬab 80,8–13; IAU 3.2/1030 f.

485 Cf. note 424 above.

486 Cf. note 421 above.

487 Cf. FagBM 2/327,16 with LéPrEM 153.

488 The sentence *wa-kāna l-muqīm li-riyāsatihī Aḥmad ibn Ilyās al-qāʾid* is not straightforward to interpret; Vernet translates "Entonces era presidente del colegio de Médicos el caid Aḥmad b. Ilyās" (VerMA 460 no. 49,3 f.), whilst the translators of Ibn Abī Uṣaybiʿa's parallel transmission settle for "(He served al-Nāṣir as physician) when Aḥmad ibn Ilyās al-Qāʾid was governor" (IAU 3.2/1030,10). The first option is over-interpretative, the second is completely evasive, but my own translation is not entirely certain either.

dignified man. al-Nāṣir—may God be pleased with him—appointed him as chief of the Court of Appeal, and [also entrusted him with] the administration of justice in Sidonia; [Muḥammad] was [further] responsible for the distribution of alms. [His life] extended into the beginning of the reign of al-Mustanṣir,[489] who appointed him as building supervisor for the expansion of the Mezquita—his name is, moreover, clearly visible ﴾١٠٩﴿ in the upper part of the prayer niche.[490] His name was also engraved on gold coins,[491] because he oversaw the Mint and Calibrations.[492] He was a knowledgeable physician. On medicine, he [wrote] a nice work which he called *Book of Forms*.[493]

50
Abū l-Walīd Muḥammad ibn Ḥusayn known as al-Kattānī[494]

[His life] extended into the end of the reign of al-Nāṣir,[495] whom he served as physician, and the beginning of the reign of al-Mustanṣir.[496] He was an elegant, generous, soft-spoken [and] noble-minded man, loved by high and low alike for his liberality in [sharing] knowledge and his charity [in helping others] at his own expense. He was not a man to be interested in money or its accumulation.

---

489 Cf. note 290 above.

490 The construction works in question refer to the expansion of the mosque's prayer hall; they began, on the order of al-Mustanṣir, already in 350/961 and were finished, according to Ṣāʿid al-Andalusī, in the year 358/969, see ṢATab 80,12 f. (who further specifies that Muḥammad ibn Tamlīkh's name "was written in gold, inlaid in a mosaic on the wall of the prayer niche, [with an inscription stating] that the construction was completed under his supervision").

491 *mithqāl*, in this context, refers to the numismatic weight of the gold dinar and, by extension, to the coin itself, cf. HiMW 1 f.

492 On the technical connotations of *amānāt*, here translated "Calibrations" (of weights and measures), cf. DoSupp 1/39a.

493 *Kitāb al-Ashkāl* (?); IAU 2.2/923,-1 only says that Muḥammad ibn Tamlīkh authored a 'Medical Book' (*Kitāb fī l-Ṭibb*).

494 Otherwise only known through Ṣāʿid al-Andalusī's and Ibn Abī Uṣaybiʿa's brief entries, both of which partly depend on Ibn Juljul's present account, cf. ṢATab 80,14 f. and IAU 3.2/1031 (*Ibn* al-Kattānī). Abū l-Walīd is not to be confused with his nephew and pupil *Abū ʿAbdallāh* Muḥammad ibn al-Ḥusayn Ibn al-Kattānī (d. ca. 421/1030), author of three medical works of which only the treatise titled *Kitāb al-Shajara* or "Book of the Tree" is preserved, see UllMed 270, GaS 3/319 f. and, for an edition with Spanish translation of the latter text, IKLib *passim*.

495 Cf. note 421 above.

496 Cf. note 290 above.

He was gentle in treating the sick, fully committed, well-informed [and] very experienced. He died of dropsy.

﴿١١٠﴾ 51
Aḥmad ibn Ḥakam ibn Ḥafṣūn[497]

He was a noble-minded, very talented [and] highly intelligent [man], a philosopher [and] somebody who knew the *Koran* by heart. He rendered medical service to al-Mustanṣir bi-llāh.[498] The chamberlain Jaʿfar[499] was the one who promoted him into a position of leadership[500]—he replaced with him [a physician] by the name of Abū ʿAbdallāh Ibn Saʿd,[501] but we are not mentioning Ibn Saʿd [in this book] because his stint was very brief and his grasp [of medicine] poor. Our Aḥmad ibn Ḥakam served as [court] physician throughout the days of Jaʿfar, yet with the death of the chamberlain[502] he was removed from the Medical Register and spent his final years in obscurity. [Aḥmad] was an eloquent speaker, a sharp theoretician, [and] well-acquainted with the terms of logic. He died of diarrhoea.

497 Otherwise only known through Ṣāʿid al-Andalusī's and Ibn Abī Uṣaybiʿa's brief entries, both of which depend on Ibn Juljul's present account, cf. ṢAṬab 80,3–7 and IAU 3.2/1033 (ibn *Ḥakīm*).

498 Cf. note 290 above.

499 Jaʿfar ibn ʿAbd al-Raḥmān *al-Ṣaqlabī* "the Slav" (ṢAṬab 80,5: *al-Sqlī*, IAU 2.2/925,5: *al-Ṣqlī*, perhaps correct *al-Ṣiqillī* "the Sicilian"?) was al-Mustanṣir's chamberlain, see FagBM 2/386 ff. with LéPrEM 65 and 106 f. The editor of Ibn Juljul's text identifies him (JulṬab 110 note 1) with the poet, chamberlain and vizier Jaʿfar ibn ʿUthmān al-Muṣḥafī, a Berber who died in prison in the year 372/982, cf. FagBM 2/391, 413 ff., 420 f. and *passim* with LéPrEM 109.

500 Here again (cf. note 488 above), the sentence *wa-kāna l-muqīm li-riyāsatihi l-ḥājib Jaʿfar* is not easy to interpret; Vernet translates "Fue jefe de la casa del chambelán Ŷaʿfar" (VerMA 460 no. 51,3), but this is hard to justify. Note in passing that Vernet also misunderstands the grammar and syntax of the Arabic clause that immediately follows the phrase in question. Ṣāʿid al-Andalusī and, after him, Ibn Abī Uṣaybiʿa omit this phrase altogether, saying instead that Aḥmad ibn Ḥakam was associated with Jaʿfar, looking after his private affairs, and that the latter introduced him to the caliph, see ṢAṬab 80,4 f. = IAU 2.2/925,5.

501 Not known otherwise.

502 The date of Jaʿfar (ibn ʿAbd al-Raḥmān's) death is not known; Jaʿfar (ibn ʿUthmān) died in 372/982.

52
Abū Bakr Aḥmad ibn Jābir[503]

He rendered medical service to al-Mustanṣir bi-llāh[504] and [kept practising until[505]] the beginning of the reign of al-Muʾayyad.[506] [Aḥmad ibn Jābir] was a mild-tempered, obliging old man, with little [interest in] high culture [but] a devout physician. The sons of al-Nāṣir[507] venerated and honoured him, knowing his due,[508] whilst the courtiers considered him a person of distinction and trustworthiness.

﴿١١١﴾ 53
Abū ʿAbd al-Malik al-Thaqafī[509]

He put the art of medicine into the service of al-Nāṣir[510] and al-Mustanṣir.[511] He was lame. There are [many] anecdotes, involving medicine, about him. al-Mustanṣir bi-llāh and al-Nāṣir (both) put him in charge of the arsenal. Towards the end of his life he became blind, due to liquid descending into his eyes.[512] He was a lettered man, familiar with the book of Euclid[513] and with the science of measurements. He was [also] a glutton for food.

He himself told me about his old times,[514] saying: "I made myself known to Najm the head falconer[515]—on festive days he always sent me twenty rams, a

503 Otherwise only known through Ibn Abī Uṣaybiʿa's account, which seems to be based on a source other than Ibn Juljul, see IAU 3.2/1033 f.

504 Cf. note 290 above.

505 Or: "lived until".

506 That is the third Umayyad caliph of Córdoba, Hishām II ibn al-Ḥakam al-Muʾayyad bi-llāh (reg. 366/976–399/1009 and, again, 400/1010–403/1013).

507 Cf. note 421 above.

508 Vernet's translation (VerMA 460 no. 52,4) of the phrase (*ʿalā*) *maʿrifat ḥaqqihī* by "le consideraban como un verdadero sabio" is wrong.

509 Otherwise only known through Ṣāʿid al-Andalusī's and Ibn Abī Uṣaybiʿa's brief entries, both of which are curtailed paraphrases of Ibn Juljul's present account, see ṢAṬab 80,16 f. (ʿAbd al-Malik al-Thaqafī) and IAU 3.2/1034 (Abū ʿAbdallāh al-Malik al-Thaqafī).

510 Cf. note 421 above.

511 Cf. note 290 above.

512 That is, cataracts.

513 This is a reference to Euclid's mathematical treatise titled *Στοιχεῖα* "Elements"; on Euclid cf. also biography **14** above.

514 Vernet's translation (VerMA 461 no. 53,6) of the phrase *ʿan zamān kāna fīhī* by "cierta vez que estuve con él" is not correct; closer but still doubtful is the translation given in IAU 3.2/1034 note 2[1], viz. "about something that happened to him".

515 That is Najm ibn Ṭarafa (cf. biography **47** above, first paragraph), who is not known otherwise.

hundred chickens and geese, and countless [other] blessings!" In the end, [Abū ʿAbd al-Malik] died of diarrhoea.[516]

﴾١١٢﴿ 54
Abū Mūsā Hārūn al-Ushūnī[517]

He was a hands-on physician.[518] He served al-Nāṣir[519] and al-Mustanṣir,[520] and looked after [their] concubines[521] and women. He was a master physician and one of their best.

55/56
Aḥmad ibn Yūnus and his brother ʿUmar the sons of Yūnus ibn Aḥmad al-Ḥarrānī[522]

They both travelled to the East during the reign of al-Nāṣir,[523] in the year 330,[524] and stayed [there] for a decade.[525] They went to Baghdad, where they studied medicine and were apprenticed to the masters, such as Thābit ibn Sinān ibn Thābit ibn Qurra,[526] with whom they read all the books of Galen; they [also] became apprentices of Ibn Waṣīf[527] [and learned from him] how to treat the eye. Then they departed to al-Andalus, where they arrived during the reign of al-Mustanṣir,[528] in the year 351.[529] ﴾١١٣﴿ They joined [the caliph] on his

516 IAU 3.2/1034,12: "of dropsy" (*istisqāʾ* instead of *ishāl*, undotted Arabic اسسسا / اسهال).

517 Otherwise only known through Ibn Abī Uṣaybiʿa's parallel account, which paraphrases (and abridges even more) that of Ibn Juljul, see IAU 3.2/1034. The designation *al-Ushūnī* refers to a native of *Osuna*, a town and district east of Seville; Vernet's and Llavero Ruiz's reading (VerMA 461 no. 54,1 and ŶulGen 101,-9) *al-Aświanī* should be emended accordingly.

518 Vernet (VerMA 461 no. 54,1) takes the phrase *khādim bi-yadihī* to mean "cirujano".

519 Cf. note 421 above.

520 Cf. note 290 above.

521 Read *lil-ḥurum*.

522 On Yūnus ibn Aḥmad al-Ḥarrānī, the father, see biography **37** above. On his sons Aḥmad (d. after 366/976) and ʿUmar (d. before 366/976) cf. also ṢATab 80,18–81,7; AbbTak 1/69f. no. 23 and 3/293f. no. 2608; QifTaʾ 395,18f. with 436,14f.; IAU 3.2/1021f.

523 Cf. note 421 above.

524 That is 942 CE.

525 But see note 529 below.

526 On him see biography **29** above.

527 On him see biography **30** above.

528 Cf. note 290 above.

529 That is 962 CE. According to the two dates specified by Ibn Juljul, the brothers stayed in the East for twenty-one years (from 330/942 to 351/962), whereas at the beginning of this paragraph he says that they stayed there for a decade—perhaps the latter specification, viz. *ʿashara* "ten", is to be emended to read *ʿishrīna* "twenty" (?).

military campaigns to San Esteban [de Gormaz][530] but left [the army when] he took them into his service as [court] physicians—he installed them in Medina Azara[531] and, wanting only those two at his disposal, excluded [most] other physicians of that time [from his service]. [When] ʿUmar fell ill with a tumour of the stomach, which withered him and led to his death, Aḥmad was left as the sole favourite of al-Mustanṣir, who moved him into his own palace in Medina Azara. [Aḥmad] was held in friendly esteem by [the caliph]: in summer, he would sit in front of him, [wearing] a thin tunic, and arrange his food—this is how close he was to the Commander of the Faithful, who [in fact] considered him loyal and trustworthy enough to look after [his] family, including the wives. [Aḥmad] was a mild-tempered, common-sensical man with a deep understanding [of medicine], thanks to the [methods of] treatment he had witnessed and [all] that he had seen with his own eyes in the East.

He himself told me [the following story], saying: "I described to the Commander of the Faithful, al-Mustanṣir bi-llāh, the well-built stalls of the cooks I had seen in Basra, the pleasing arrangement of the food which was placed in porcelain vessels covered with glass lids, the servants standing ready with towels and [water] jugs, and the floors [tiled] with multicoloured marble of exquisite beauty. Another day, al-Mustanṣir rode out from [Medina] Azara to Córdoba, I in his retinue. When he came to the market,[532] [and there to] the quarter of the cooks, he noticed the hot ashes and glowing embers[533] in which the fatty meat was being roasted, and he longly contemplated them. Back in the palace, he realized I was not by his side and sent for me. He said: 'O Aḥmad! How far are these ashes and embers from those porcelain vessels they have in Basra!', and he sniggered about it. Then he said: 'What is in these ashes and embers?' And [when] I replied: 'Limbs and grease, O Commander of the Faithful', he let out an astonished laugh".

[Aḥmad] was in charge of running the palace pharmacy, which was quite unique in its kind—twelve young Slavs[534] he had working there to cook the potions and to prepare the electuaries. He asked for and was granted permis-

---

530 Arabic *Shant Istibyn* (استبين < *استبان*?), an important (Christian) town in the province of Soria, central Spain.

531 Medina Azara, a catalanized form of Arabic *Madīnat al-Zahrāʾ* "the Radiant City", was a fortified palace-city and seat of government ca. 5 km northwest of Córdoba; the bulk of the city's construction was completed under the caliph al-Nāṣir, between the years 325/936 and 329/940, but building works continued in various phases well into the reign of his successor al-Mustanṣir, see LéPrEM 225–231 and OcJiMZ *passim*.

532 Read *al-mudy*. Cf. JulṬab 114 note 9 with ŶulGen 128 note 187 (ibid. 103,7 emend *almudi*).

533 Read *al-malal*.

534 Cf. note 478 above.

sion by the Commander of the Faithful to give some of these [medicines] to poor and sick people who needed them. [Aḥmad] was well-acquainted with simple drugs [and] a skilled maker of potions and electuaries, [capable of] treating whatever he was presented with.[535] For eye [diseases] he knew precious therapies, and [many] stories are still being told about him in Córdoba. He never exempted wealthy people from sending him money in return for treatment, but he always offered his [medical] skill for free to a friend, a neighbour or a pauper. al-Muʾayyad bi-llāh[536] appointed him chief of the police and inspector of the public market. [Aḥmad] had a speech impediment [and] his handwriting was very bad, with the letters all jumbled up. He died of quartan fever and diarrhoea.[537]

﴿١١٥﴾ 57
Muḥammad ibn ʿAbdūn al-Jabalī al-ʿAdadī[538]

He travelled to the East in the year 347[539] and went to Basra, without visiting Baghdad. He [then] directed himself to the city of Fusṭāṭ [in Egypt], where he

535 The phrase *muʿālij* ^{an} *li-mā waqafa ʿalayhī* has been translated by Vernet "atendía a todo aquél que se le presentaba" (VerMA 462,16), whilst the translators of Ibn Abī Uṣaybiʿa's parallel transmission have "which he employed for the appropriate treatments" (IAU 3.2/1022,4f.).

536 Cf. note 506 above.

537 ŶulGen 128 note 189 considers this to be malaria, saying: "Se trata de la malaria (paludismo cuartano), siendo uno de sus síntomas la disentería" (?).

538 Muḥammad ibn ʿAbdūn, a physician, mathematician and logician from Córdoba who died after the year 366/976, see UllMed 274 note 2, GaS 3/303 and DjJab *passim*. There is some confusion regarding the last element of Muḥammad ibn ʿAbdūn's name: the editor of Ibn Juljul's text, Fuʾād Sayyid, and (after him) Juan Vernet read *al-ʿAdadī*, lit. "the Numberman" (scil. mathematician), see JulṬab 115 ad 57 = VerMA 462 note 157; Manfred Ullmann, Fuat Sezgin and Ahmed Djebbar read *al-ʿUdhrī*, that is a member or descendant of the Arab tribe of ʿUdhra, see UllMed, GaS and DjJab locs cit.; and the editors/translators of Ibn Abī Uṣaybiʿa's parallel transmission read *al-ʿIdwī*, referring to an explanation given in DoSupp 2/105b (viz. "d'outre-mer, qui vient du nord de l'Afrique"), and on the grounds that Muḥammad ibn ʿAbdūn returned to Spain via North Africa and across the Strait of Gibraltar, see IAU 3.2/1035 note 1. The underlying Arabic forms of that name (العدوي / العذري / العددي et al.) are indeed open to several interpretations, and my adopted reading *al-ʿAdadī* is just as likely as *al-ʿUdhrī*; on the other hand, the reading *al-ʿIdwī*, though semantically sound, seems to me a rather far-fetched choice, not least because it could (and should) have equally been applied to a whole range of Andalusian travellers who returned from abroad in precisely this way.

539 That is 958 CE.

became head of the hospital.[540] He returned to al-Andalus in the year 360,[541] and served as [court] physician to al-Mustanṣir bi-llāh[542] and al-Muʾayyad bi-llāh.[543] Before he practised medicine, he taught arithmetic in al-Andalus.[544] [He was] a skilled, well-versed and seasoned physician.

﴿١١٦﴾ I have now, O Sire,[545] mentioned all that I know for certain and that fell within my reach, regarding famous sages and physicians of indubitable [reputation], from the time of Adam—peace be upon him—down to our present era, which is the time of al-Muʾayyad bi-llāh,[546] in the realm of al-Andalus. We have mentioned those among them who lived in the East and [those who lived in] the West, but omitted conspicuous Easterners between the reign of al-Rāḍī[547] and the days of al-Ṭāʾiʿ li-llāh,[548] because this would have exceeded our grasp as well as our intention—under those declining regimes which were infiltrated by the power of the Daylamites and the Turks, who are indifferent to knowledge, no truly outstanding man arose who may deserve to be noticed for his mastery or who is renowned for his contributions:[549] sages appear only in states whose rulers seek wisdom. [Instead] we concentrated on famous, well-known [and] accessible [men] from our homeland of al-Andalus, [who lived] under the guidance of leaders—kings, sons of kings—that pursued knowledge and strove for wisdom. We [further] narrowed our focus on naming those [among them] who served [the court], but not such of their contemporaries as were no match for them[550] nor occupied an equally [import-

540 This is a reference to the hospital founded in the year 259/873 by the erstwhile governor and later practically independent ruler of Egypt, Aḥmad ibn Ṭūlūn (d. 270/884), see DuBīm *passim*. Fusṭāṭ, originally established as a military camp in the course of the Arab conquest of Egypt, gradually developed into a city, which became and remained the capital of Muslim Egypt until the foundation of Cairo in 358/969. It is possible that Muḥammad ibn ʿAbdūn left Egypt in the wake of the Fāṭimid invasion of the country.

541 That is 971 CE.

542 Cf. note 290 above.

543 Cf. note 506 above.

544 ṢAṬab 81,12 f. and, after him, IAU 2.2/926,-2 f. say: "… he taught arithmetic and geometry, and (wrote) a nice book (titled) 'On Fractions' (*Fī l-Taksīr*)".

545 Cf. note 1 above.

546 Cf. note 506 above.

547 That is the twentieth ʿAbbāsid caliph Abū l-ʿAbbās Aḥmad (or Muḥammad) ibn Jaʿfar al-Rāḍī bi-llāh (reg. 322/934–329/940).

548 That is the twenty-fourth ʿAbbāsid caliph Abū Bakr ʿAbd al-Karīm ibn al-Faḍl al-Ṭāʾiʿ li-llāh (reg. 363/974–381/991).

549 Note, however, that Ibn Juljul *does* mention some 'Easterners' who lived well into the time of al-Rāḍī, see biographies **29**, **30** and **31** above.

550 Read *yuwāzihim* (instead of *yuwāzīhim*).

ant] position, worthy of being dealt with at any length. Thus I recounted [the formers'] circumstances and merits, as well as anecdotes and [other] news about them that have come to light, choosing quality over quantity so as not to exhaust the reader's patience, and to make it easier for the mind to retain [the information]—for overmuch talking is hard to bear. So let it be enough that we disclosed and narrated the best [aspects] of everything in due brevity!

At the end of this epistle, O Sire, I am [also] recounting the course of my own life, the education I received, and how I searched [for knowledge], always aiming at the truth—God is the witness of what I say! I felt that [my] epistle could not be left without such [an appendix], seeing what memorable events and convenient revelations it contains.[551] And to God I turn for help.

---

551 It is a highly regrettable fact that the unique Arabic manuscript of Ibn Juljul's *Ṭabaqāt* lacks these final autobiographical remarks—cf. p. 7 above with note 38.

Addendum

I would like to take this opportunity and put on record a small number of philological observations which Manfred Ullmann kindly communicated to me in a personal letter dated 24 October 2022. These observations concern my edition and translation of ʿAlī ibn Sahl al-Ṭabarī's so-called *Indian Books*, published by Brill in August 2022 as volume 121 of the series "Islamic Philosophy, Theology and Science" (cf. bibliography s.n. ṬabIB). Ullmann's learned remarks are highly unlikely to ever appear in print elsewhere, and it would be a shame not to share them. They are reproduced here in Ullmann's exact words, with the exception of bibliographical sigla, which have been adjusted to the conventions used in the present book and can be found in the general bibliography below; page numbers (in boldface) refer to ṬabIB, the work in question; square brackets indicate additions on my part. Here is Ullmann:

82,7 f. ist *ṭuḥāl* zu vokalisieren, s. WgaÜ S 2/317 s.v. *σπληνιάω*, also "disease" gehört nicht in Klammern; dasselbe gilt für *baṭan* "belly(ache)", nicht in Klammern, s. GALex 2/325 (für *διάρροια* bzw. *δυσεντερία*) | **82**,10 *yuṭayyibu l-nafasa* "macht den Atem wohlriechend" | **89** Anm. 86 *al-sūdāniyyu* ist bei Arist[oteles] H[istoria] A[nimalium] 617b,26 = *ψάρος* [Star], s. WgaÜ 779 | **98** Anm. 97 Zu *kusb* vgl. WkaS 1/171b | **110**,3 *iltāma bi-hī* heißt "sich mit etw. vereinigen, verbinden, mit etw. zusammenhängen", vgl. WkaS 2/1812a; aber was heißt "er soll kein störrisches Reittier besteigen und auch nicht das, was damit zusammenhängt"? M[eines] E[rachtens] ist mit den Varianten zu lesen *wa-lā yaghtarru … bi-mā yutashāʾamu bi-hī* "er soll sich auch nicht täuschen lassen durch das, was als übles Vorzeichen betrachtet wird" [this proposition, however, cannot be reconciled with the Sanskrit sources]; der dazwischen geschaltete Satz *wa-lā yarkabu min al-dawābbi ṣaʿban* steht wohl nicht an der richtigen Stelle [?] | **110**,5 *wa-lā tufāriquhu l-aḥjāru llatī yudfaʿu bi-hā l-siḥr* heißt "er soll stets Steine, mit denen Zauber abgewehrt wird, bei sich haben" (vgl. Anm. 130) [this actually corresponds to my own translation] | **112**,1 *wa-yujarriʾuhū ʿalayhī* "and emboldens the enemy *against him*" | **138**,1 Zu *nayṭ* plur. *anyāṭ* vgl. JawTāj 1/568,5 f. *wa-l-niyāṭu: ʿirqun ʿulliqa bi-hi l-qalbu min al-watīni fa-idhā quṭiʿa māta ṣāḥibuhū, wa-huwa l-nayṭu ayḍan* (= FrLex s.v., aber die Wurzel ist *nwṭ*) | **142** Anm. 187 Zu *qāriʿa* vgl. grundlegend UllBei 207–210 (nr. CXVI) | **148**,4 Das berühmte *καρφολογέω* bei H[i]p[pocrates] Progn[osticum] 4, s. WgaÜ 328 | **150**,4 *iltazamat waladahā* "sie umarmt ihr Kind, drückt es an sich", s. WkaS 2/562a | **154**,6 ist zitiert bei UllFlü nr. 582 | **172**,1 *ʿūd al-alanjūj* vgl. WkaS 2/226a | **174**,4 *fī waqti jaryi l-māʾi fī l-ʿūd* heißt "zur Zeit, wenn der Saft im Holz aufsteigt" | **178**,4 *yuṭayyibu l-nafasa*

© KONINKLIJKE BRILL NV, LEIDEN, 2023 | DOI:10.1163/9789004682238_004

"macht den Atem wohlriechend" | *al-malīla* heißt "feverish heat" bzw. "intense thirst", vgl. AzTah 15/352a,15f. *yuqālu: bi-hī malīlatun wa-mulālun wa-dhālika ḥarāratun yajiduhā* | Was ist *al-ibrada*? Lies vielleicht *al-ibriya* = *πίτυρον* [Kopfkleie, Hautschorf], s. WgaÜ S 2/119 | 184,3 lies *illā khurrija* | 206,6 Zu *lumjatun* "Happen, Bissen" vgl. WkaS 2/1340a, wo der Plural *lumajātun* nicht belegt ist ‖ Sed haec hactenus!

Bibliography

This bibliography contains *cited* literature only.

AbbTak = Muḥammad ibn ʿAbdallāh Ibn al-Abbār, *al-Takmila li-kitāb al-Ṣila*, 1–4, ed. B. ʿAwwād Maʿrūf, Tūnis (Dār al-Gharb al-Islāmī) 1432/2011 (Silsilat al-Tarājim al-Andalusiyya 7).

AdKin = P. Adamson, "al-Kindī", in: *EI*³ [q.v.] s.n.

ÁlMiBD = C. Álvarez Millán, "Medical Anecdotes in Ibn Juljul's Biographical Dictionary", in: *Suhayl* 4 (2004), pp. 141–158.

ÁlMiIŶ = C. Álvarez Millán, "Ibn Ŷulŷul, Abū Dawūd Sulaymān b. Ḥassān", in: *Diccionario Biográfico Español*, vol. 27, Madrid (Real Academia de la Historia) 2009, pp. 66–69.

AltIS = A. Altmann, "Isḥāḳ b. Sulaymān al-Isrāʾīlī", in: *EI*² [q.v.] s.n.

AMMin¹ = *Alberti Magni Philosophorum Maximi De Mineralibus Libri Quinque*, Augusta Vindelicorum (Sigismund Grimm & Marcus Vuyrsung) 1519.

AMMin² = *Albertus Magnus. Book of Minerals*, tr. D. Wyckoff, Oxford (Oxford University Press) 1967.

AMpo = E. Acampora-Michel, *Liber de pomo / Buch vom Apfel*, Frankfurt am Main (Vittorio Klostermann) 2001.

AnaTA = G.C. Anawati, "Textes arabes anciens édités en Égypte au cours des années 1955 et 1956", in: *Mélanges de l'Institut Dominicain d'Études Orientales du Caire* 3 (1956), pp. 259–348.

AncGS = C. D'Ancona, "Greek Sources in Arabic and Islamic Philosophy", in: *Stanford Encyclopedia of Philosophy* [plato.stanford.edu/archives/spr2022/entries/arabic-islamic-greek].

ʿAsTT = Aḥmad ibn ʿAlī Ibn Ḥajar al-ʿAsqalānī, *Tahdhīb al-tahdhīb*, 1–4, ed. I. al-Zaybaq and ʿA. Murshid, [Bayrūt] (Muʾassasat al-Risāla) 1416/1995.

AzTah = Muḥammad ibn Aḥmad al-Azharī, *Tahdhīb al-lugha*, 1–15, ed. ʿAbd al-Salām Hārūn, al-Qāhira (al-Dār al-Miṣriyya lil-Taʾlīf wa-l-Tarjama) 1384/1964–1387/1967.

BadUṣ = ʿAbd al-Raḥmān Badawī, *Kitāb al-Siyāsa fī tadbīr al-riyāsa al-maʿrūf bi-Sirr al-asrār*, in: *al-Uṣūl al-yūnāniyya lil-naẓariyyāt al-siyāsiyya fī l-islām*, al-Qāhira (Maktabat al-Nahḍa al-Miṣriyya) 1954 (Dirāsāt Islāmiyya 15), pp. 65–171.

BaGal = P. Bachmann, *Galens Abhandlung darüber, daß der vorzügliche Arzt Philosoph sein muß*, Göttingen (Vandenhoeck & Ruprecht) 1965 (Nachrichten der Akademie der Wissenschaften in Göttingen, Philologisch-Historische Klasse 1).

BaGuEM = M.-G. Balty-Guesdon, *Médecins et hommes de sciences en Espagne musulmane (IIᵉ/VIIIᵉ–Vᵉ/XIᵉ siècles)*, Thèse de Doctorat, Université Paris-III, 1992 (unpublished) [microfiche available from *Atelier National de Reproduction des Thèses*, Université de Lille, ref.-no. 92PA030127].

BarGal = *Galeni De Optimo Docendi Genere* [and] *Exhortatio ad Medicinam* (*Protrepticus*), ed. A. Barigazzi, Berlin (Akademie-Verlag) 1991 (Corpus Medicorum Graecorum 5/1-1).

BashṢi = Khalaf ibn ʿAbd al-Malik Ibn Bashkuwāl, *al-Ṣila fī taʾrīkh aʾimmat al-Andalus wa-ʿulamāʾihim wa-muḥaddithīhim wa-fuqahāʾihim wa-udabāʾihim*, 1–2, ed. B. ʿAwwād Maʿrūf, Tūnis (Dār al-Gharb al-Islāmī) 1431/2010 (Silsilat al-Tarājim al-Andalusiyya 5).

BergGÜ = G. Bergsträsser, *Ḥunain ibn Isḥāq über die syrischen und arabischen Galen-Übersetzungen*, Leipzig (Brockhaus) 1925 (Abhandlungen für die Kunde des Morgenlandes 17/2).

BHDuw = Abū l-Faraj Ibn al-ʿIbrī (Barhebraeus), *Mukhtaṣar taʾrīkh al-duwal*, ed. A. Ṣāliḥānī, Bayrūt (al-Maṭbaʿa al-Kāthūlīkiyya) 1890.

BlaAH = K. van Bladel, *The Arabic Hermes. From Pagan Sage to Prophet of Science*, Oxford (Oxford University Press) 2009 (Oxford Studies in Late Antiquity).

BoAṢM = C.E. Bosworth, "Abū Ṣāleḥ Manṣūr", in: *EIr* [q.v.] s.n.

BoViIḲ = J. Bosch-Vilá, "Ibn al-Ḳūṭiyya", in: *EI*² [q.v.] s.n.

CarSī = M.G. Carter, "Sībawayhi", in: *EI*² [q.v.] s.n.

ChMan = P. Chalmeta, "al-Manṣūr", in: *EI*² [q.v.] s.n.

ChMuw = P. Chalmeta, "Muwallad", in: *EI*² [q.v.] s.n.

CouCC = S. Coughlin, "Cohesive Causes in Ancient Greek Philosophy and Medicine", in: *Holism in Ancient Medicine and its Reception*, ed. C. Thumiger, Leiden–Boston (Brill) 2021 (Studies in Ancient Medicine 53), pp. 237–267.

CPPL = M. Rosser-Owen, *Articulating the Ḥijāba: Cultural Patronage and Political Legitimacy in al-Andalus. The ʿĀmirid Regency c. 970–1010 AD*, Leiden–Boston (Brill) 2022 (Handbook of Oriental Studies, Section One, The Near and Middle East 156).

ḌabbBu = Aḥmad ibn Yaḥyā al-Ḍabbī, *Bughyat al-multamis fī taʾrīkh rijāl ahl al-Andalus*, ed. F. Codera and J. Ribera, Madrid (Rojas) 1884 (Bibliotheca Arabico-Hispana 3).

DaiOr = H. Daiber, "Orosius' *Historiae adversus paganos* in arabischer Überlieferung", in: *Tradition and Re-Interpretation in Jewish and Early Christian Literature. Essays in Honour of Jürgen C.H. Lebram*, ed. J.W. van Henten et al., Leiden (E.J. Brill) 1986 (Studia Post-Biblica 36), pp. 202–249.

DalMM = O. El Daly, *Egyptology: The Missing Millennium. Ancient Egypt in Medieval Arabic Writings*, London–NewYork (Routledge) 2009 (University College London, Institute of Archaeology Publications 33).

DaNuʿ = F. Dachraoui, "al-Nuʿmān", in: *EI*² [q.v.] s.n.

DarOG = C. Daremberg, *Œuvres anatomiques, physiologiques et médicales de Galien. Traduites sur les textes imprimés et manuscrits, accompagnées de sommaires, de notes, de planches et d'une table des matières, précédées d'une introduction ou étude biographique, littéraire et scientifique sur Galien*, 1–2, Paris (J.B. Baillière) 1854–1856.

DhaTI = Muḥammad ibn Aḥmad al-Dhahabī, *Taʾrīkh al-islām wa-wafayāt al-mashāhīr wa-l-aʿlām*, 1–17, ed. B. ʿAwwād Maʿrūf, Bayrūt (Dār al-Gharb al-Islāmī) 1424/2003.

DietIDj = A. Dietrich, "Ibn Djuldjul", in: *EI*² [q.v.] s.n.

DietMā = A. Dietrich, "Māsardjawayh", in: *EI*² [q.v.] s.n.

DietMM = A. Dietrich, *Die Ergänzung Ibn Ǧulǧul's zur Materia medica des Dioskurides*, Göttingen (Vandenhoeck & Ruprecht) 1993 (Abhandlungen der Akademie der Wissenschaften in Göttingen, Philologisch-Historische Klasse, Dritte Folge 202).

DioMM = *Pedanii Dioscuridis Anazarbei De Materia Medica Libri Quinque*, 1–3, ed. M. Wellmann, Berolini (Weidmann) 1906–1914.

DjJab = A. Djebbar, "Ibn ʿAbdūn al-Jabalī", in: *EI*³ [q.v.] s.n.

DoFih = B. Dodge, *The Fihrist of al-Nadīm. A Tenth-Century Survey of Muslim Culture*, 1–2, NewYork–London (Columbia University Press) 1970 (Records of Civilization 83).

DoHis = R. Dozy, *Histoire des musulmans d'Espagne jusqu'à la conquête de l'Andalousie par les Almoravides (711–1110)*, 1–4, Leyde (E.J. Brill) 1861.

DoSupp = R. Dozy, *Supplément aux dictionnaires arabes*, 1–2, Leide–Paris (E.J. Brill & Maisonneuve Frères) 1927².

DuBīm = D.M. Dunlop, "Bīmāristān", in: *EI*² [q.v.] s.n.

DucIs = J.-C. Ducène, "al-Bakrī et les *Étymologies* d'Isidore de Séville", in: *Journal Asiatique* 297 (2009), pp. 379–397.

DunTr = D.M. Dunlop, "The Translations of al-Biṭrīq and Yaḥyā (Yūḥannā) b. al-Biṭrīq", in: *Journal of the Royal Asiatic Society of Great Britain and Ireland* no. 3/4 (1959), pp. 140–150.

EDG = R. Beekes with the assistance of L. van Beek, *Etymological Dictionary of Greek*, 1–2, Leiden–Boston (Brill) 2010 (Leiden Indo-European Etymological Dictionary Series 10).

EI² = *The Encyclopaedia of Islam. Second Edition*, 1–12, ed. C.E. Bosworth et al., Leiden (Brill) 1960–2004 [referenceworks.brillonline.com/browse/encyclopaedia-of-islam-2].

EI³ = *Encyclopaedia of Islam. Three*, 1—, ed. K. Fleet et al., Leiden–Boston (Brill) 2007— [referenceworks.brillonline.com/browse/encyclopaedia-of-islam-3].

EIr = *Encyclopædia Iranica*, 1—, ed. E. Yarshater [then] E.L. Daniel et al., London [then] NewYork [then] Leiden (Routledge & Kegan Paul [then] Encyclopædia Iranica Foundation [then] Koninklijke Brill) 1985—[iranicaonline.org].

EtyIs = *The Etymologies of Isidore of Seville*, tr. S.A. Barney, W.J. Lewis, J.A. Beach and O. Berghof, with the collaboration of M. Hall, Cambridge (Cambridge University Press) 2006.

FagBM = *Histoire de l'Afrique et de l'Espagne intitulée al-Bayano'l-Mogrib [d'Ibn ʿIdhārī]*, 1–2, tr. E. Fagnan, Alger (Imprimerie Orientale Pierre Fontana) 1901–1904.

FarTa' = ʿAbdallāh ibn Muḥammad Ibn al-Faraḍī, *Taʾrīkh ʿulamāʾ al-Andalus*, 1–2, ed.

B. ʿAwwād Maʿrūf, Tūnis (Dār al-Gharb al-Islāmī) 1429/2008 (Silsilat al-Tarājim al-Andalusiyya 1).

FiCG = G. Fichtner et al., *Corpus Galenicum. Bibliographie der galenischen und pseudogalenischen Werke* [cmg.bbaw.de/fileadmin/Webdateien/Dateien/Galen-Bibliographie_2019-01.pdf].

FiCH = G. Fichtner et al., *Corpus Hippocraticum. Bibliographie der hippokratischen und pseudohippokratischen Werke* [cmg.bbaw.de/fileadmin/Webdateien/Dateien/Hippokrates-Bibliographie_2016-12.pdf].

ForʿAS = M. Forcada, "ʿArīb b. Saʿīd al-Qurṭūbī [*sic*]", in: *EI*[3] [q.v.] s.n.

ForBC = M. Forcada, "Biografías de científicos", in: *Biografías y género biográfico en el occidente islámico*, ed. M.L. Ávila and M. Marín, Madrid (Consejo Superior de Investigaciones Científicas) 1997 (Estudios Onomástico-Biográficos de al-Ándalus 8), pp. 201–248.

FordAP = A. Ford, *Aristotle as Poet. The Song for Hermias and its Contexts*, Oxford (Oxford University Press) 2011.

FrLex = G.W. Freytag, *Lexicon Arabico-Latinum*, 1–4, Halis Saxonum (C.A. Schwetschke) 1830–1837.

GaL = C. Brockelmann, *Geschichte der arabischen Litteratur*, 1–2, Leiden (E.J. Brill) 1943–1949[2], *Supplements* 1–3, Leiden (E.J. Brill) 1937–1942.

GALex = *A Greek and Arabic Lexicon (GALex). Materials for a Dictionary of the Mediaeval Translations from Greek into Arabic*, 1—, ed. R. Arnzen, G. Endress and D. Gutas with the assistance of G.J. Moseley, Leiden–Boston (Brill) 1992— (Handbook of Oriental Studies, Section One, The Near and Middle East 11).

GarIŶ = I. Garijo Galán, "Ibn Ŷulŷul, Sulaymān", in: *Biblioteca de al-Andalus*, vol. 6, Almería (Fundación Ibn Tufayl de Estudios Árabes) 2009, pp. 163–166.

GarLib = *Ibn Ŷulŷul. Libro de la explicación de los nombres de los medicamentos simples tomados del libro de Dioscórides*, ed. and tr. I. Garijo Galán, Córdoba (Universidad de Córdoba) 1992.

GarOb = I. Garijo Galán, *La obra científica de Ibn Ŷulŷul*, Tesis Doctoral, Universidad de Córdoba, 1991 (unpublished).

GarTra[1] = *Ibn Ŷulŷul. Tratado sobre los medicamentos de la tríaca*, ed. and tr. I. Garijo Galán, Córdoba (Universidad de Córdoba) 1992.

GarTra[2] = *Ibn Ŷulŷul. Tratado octavo, mencionamos en él lo que Dioscórides no cita en su libro*, ed. and tr. I. Garijo Galán, Córdoba (Universidad de Córdoba) 1992.

GaS = F. Sezgin, *Geschichte des arabischen Schrifttums*, 1–17, Leiden (E.J. Brill) 1967–1984 [then] Frankfurt am Main (Institut für Geschichte der arabisch-islamischen Wissenschaften) 2000–2015.

GayHis = *The History of the Mohammedan Dynasties in Spain. Extracted from the Nafhu-t-tíb min ghosni-l-Andalusi-r-rattíb wa táríkh Lisánu-d-Dín Ibni-l-Khattíb, by Ahmed ibn Mohammed al-Makkarí, a Native of Telemsán*, 1–2, tr. P. de Gayangos, London (The Royal Asiatic Society of Great Britain and Ireland) 1840–1843.

GiṬab = C. Gilliot, "Ṭabaḳāt", in: EI² [q.v.] s.n.

GOO = *Claudii Galeni Opera Omnia*, 1–20, ed. and tr. [into Latin] C.G. Kühn, Lipsiae (Car[olus] Cnobloch) 1821–1833 (Medicorum Graecorum Opera Quae Exstant).

GoRā = L.E. Goodman, "al-Rāzī", in: EI² [q.v.] s.n.

GueṬab = M.-G. Guesdon, "Les *Ṭabaqāt al-aṭibbā' wa l-ḥukamā'* d'Ibn Ǧulǧul: une condamnation du régime 'āmiride", in: *Cahiers d'Onomastique Arabe* (1988–1992), pp. 49–59.

GuGT = D. Gutas, *Greek Thought, Arabic Culture. The Graeco-Arabic Translation Movement in Baghdad and Early 'Abbāsid Society (2nd–4th/8th–10th Centuries)*, London–NewYork (Routledge) 1998.

GuGWL = D. Gutas, *Greek Wisdom Literature in Arabic Translation*, New Haven (American Oriental Society) 1975 (American Oriental Series 60).

HámRa = A.P. Hámori, "Ibn 'Abd Rabbih", in: EI³ [q.v.] s.n.

HaPAL = D.N. Hasse, "Plato arabico-latinus: Philosophy–Wisdom Literature–Occult Sciences", in: *The Platonic Tradition in the Middle Ages. A Doxographic Approach*, ed. S. Gersh and M. Hoenen, Berlin–NewYork (Walter de Gruyter) 2002, pp. 31–65.

HawSW = G.R. Hawting, "Sa'd b. Abī Waḳḳāṣ", in: EI² [q.v.] s.n.

HieCh = *Die Chronik des Hieronymus / Hieronymi Chronicon*, ed. R. Helm, Berlin (Akademie-Verlag) 1956 (Die Griechischen Christlichen Schriftsteller der Ersten Jahrhunderte 47 = Eusebius Werke 7).

HiḲL = D. Hill, "Ḳuṣtā [*sic*] b. Lūḳā", in: EI² [q.v.] s.n.

HiMW = W. Hinz, *Measures and Weights in the Islamic World*, tr. M.I. Marcinkowski, Kuala Lumpur (International Institute of Islamic Thought and Civilization) 2003.

ḤumJM = Muḥammad ibn Fattūḥ al-Ḥumaydī, *Jadhwat al-muqtabas fī dhikr wulāt al-Andalus*, ed. Rawḥiyya al-Suwayfī, Bayrūt (Dār al-Kutub al-'Ilmiyya) 1417/1997.

IAU = *A Literary History of Medicine: The 'Uyūn al-anbā' fī ṭabaqāt al-aṭibbā' of Ibn Abī Uṣaybi'ah*, 1–3 [in 5 vols], ed. and tr. E. Savage-Smith, S. Swain, G.J. van Gelder et al., Leiden–Boston (Brill) 2020 (Handbook of Oriental Studies, Section One, The Near and Middle East 134).

IdIDj = H.R. Idris, "Ibn al-D̲jazzār", in: EI² [q.v.] s.n.

IḤMus = Aḥmad ibn Muḥammad Ibn Ḥanbal, *al-Musnad*, 1–19, ed. A.M. Shākir and Ḥ.A. al-Zayn, al-Qāhira (Dār al-Ḥadīth) 1416/1995.

IḤRis = 'Alī ibn Aḥmad Ibn Ḥazm al-Qurṭubī, *Risāla fī Faḍl al-Andalus wa-dhikr rijālihā*, in: MaqqNṬ [q.v.] 2/108–121.

IḤṬawq = 'Alī ibn Aḥmad Ibn Ḥazm al-Qurṭubī, *Ṭawq al-ḥamāma fī l-ulfa wa-l-ullāf*, ed. I. 'Abbās, Bayrūt (al-Mu'assasa al-'Arabiyya lil-Dirāsāt wa-l-Nashr) 1987² (Rasā'il Ibn Ḥazm al-Andalusī 1).

IKhWaf = Aḥmad ibn Muḥammad Ibn Khallikān, *Wafayāt al-a'yān wa-anbā' abnā' al-zamān*, 1–2, Būlāq 1310[/1892].

IKLib = *El "Libro del Árbol" de Ibn al-Kattānī. Un tratado médico andalusí*, ed. and tr.

J. Coullaut Cordero and C. Vázquez de Benito, Salamanca (Ediciones Universidad Salamanca) 2017 (Historia de la Medicina 19).

InkBu = B. Inksetter, "Ibn Bukhtīshūʿ Family", in: *EI*³ [q.v.] s.n.

InkḤā = B. Inksetter, "al-Ḥārith b. Kalada", in: *EI*³ [q.v.] s.n.

IQNab = Muḥammad ibn Abī Bakr Ibn Qayyim al-Jawziyya, *al-Ṭibb al-nabawī*, ed. ʿAbd al-Ghanī ʿAbd al-Khāliq et al., Bayrūt (Dār al-Fikr) 1957.

IQRaw = Muḥammad ibn Abī Bakr Ibn Qayyim al-Jawziyya, *Rawḍat al-muḥibbīn wa-nuzhat al-mushtāqīn*, facs. ed., Dimashq (Maṭbaʿat al-Taraqqī) 1349/1930.

IsEty = *Isidori Hispalensis Episcopi Etymologiarum sive Originum libri XX*, 1–2, ed. W.M. Lindsay, Oxonii (Clarendon Press) 1911 (Scriptorum Classicorum Bibliotheca Oxoniensis).

IskGal = *Galen on Examinations by which the Best Physicians are Recognized*, ed. and tr. A.Z. Iskandar, Berlin (Akademie-Verlag) 1988 (Corpus Medicorum Graecorum, Supplementum Orientale 4).

ITAk = J.T. Irvine and O. Temkin, "Who was Akīlāōs? A Problem in Medical Historiography", in: *Bulletin of the History of Medicine* 77 (2003), pp. 12–24.

ʿIyTM = al-Qāḍī ʿIyāḍ ibn Mūsā al-Sibtī, *Tartīb al-madārik wa-taqrīb al-masālik li-maʿrifat aʿlām madhhab Mālik*, 1–8, ed. M. b. Tāwīt al-Ṭanjī et al., [Tangier] (Wizārat al-Awqāf wa-l-Shuʾūn al-Islāmiyya) 1403/1983².

JanNMD = *Marwān ibn Janāḥ: On the Nomenclature of Medicinal Drugs (Kitāb al-Talkhīṣ), with special reference to the Ibero-Romance terminology*, 1–2, ed., tr. and comm. G. Bos, F. Käs, M. Lübke and G. Mensching, Leiden–Boston (Brill) 2020 (Islamic History and Civilization 170).

JawTāj = Ismāʿīl ibn Ḥammād al-Jawharī, *Tāj al-lugha wa-ṣiḥāḥ al-ʿarabiyya*, 1–2, Būlāq 1282[/1865].

JRKin = J. Jolivet and R. Rashed, "al-Kindī", in: *EI*² [q.v.] s.n.

JulṬab = Sulaymān ibn Ḥassān Ibn Juljul, *Ṭabaqāt al-aṭibbāʾ wa-l-ḥukamāʾ / Les Générations des médecins et des sages*, ed. F. Sayyid, Le Caire (Imprimerie de l'Institut Français d'Archéologie Orientale) 1955 (Publications de l'Institut Français d'Archéologie Orientale du Caire, Textes et Traductions d'Auteurs Orientaux 10).

JuNB = F. Justi, *Iranisches Namenbuch*, Marburg (N.G. Elwert) 1895.

KaCB = O. Kahl, *The Sanskrit, Syriac and Persian Sources in the Comprehensive Book of Rhazes*, Leiden–Boston (Brill) 2015 (Islamic Philosophy, Theology and Science, Texts and Studies 93).

KaeByz = W.E. Kaegi, *Byzantium and the Early Islamic Conquests*, Cambridge (Cambridge University Press) 1992.

KinAq = *The Medical Formulary or Aqrābādhīn of al-Kindī*, ed. (facsimile), tr. and comm. M. Levey, Madison–Milwaukee–London (The University of Wisconsin Press) 1966 (Publications in Medieval Science).

KMBah = Dj. Khaleghi-Motlagh, "Bahman (2) Son of Esfandīār", in: *EIr* [q.v.] s.n.

LaLex = E.W. Lane, *An Arabic-English Lexicon*, 1–8, London–Edinburgh (Williams & Norgate) 1863–1893.

LéPrEM = É. Lévi-Provençal, *L'Espagne musulmane au x*[e] *siècle. Institutions et vie sociale*, Paris (Maisonneuve & Larose) 2002 (reprint).

LongIJ = M. Long, "Ibn Juljūl [*sic*]", in: *The Oxford Encyclopedia of Philosophy, Science, and Technology in Islam*, 1–2, ed. I. Kalin, Oxford (Oxford University Press) 2014.

LSDic = C.T. Lewis and C. Short, *A New Latin Dictionary*, NewYork–Oxford (Harper & Brothers with Clarendon Press) 1891.

LSLex = H.G. Liddell and R. Scott, *A Greek-English Lexicon*, NewYork–Chicago–Cincinnati (American Book Company) 1897[8].

ManSA = M. Manzalaoui, "The Pseudo-Aristotelian *Kitāb Sirr al-Asrār*. Facts and Problems", in: *Oriens* 23–24 (1974), pp. 147–257.

MaqqNṬ = Aḥmad ibn Muḥammad al-Maqqarī, *Nafḥ al-ṭīb min ghuṣn al-Andalus al-raṭīb wa-dhikr wazīrihā Lisān al-Dīn Ibn al-Khaṭīb / Analectes sur l'histoire et la littérature des Arabes d'Espagne*, 1–2 [in 4 vols], ed. R. Dozy, G. Dugat, L. Krehl and W. Wright, Leyde (E.J. Brill) 1855–1859.

MarrDh = Muḥammad Ibn ʿAbd al-Malik al-Marrākushī, *al-Dhayl wa-l-takmila li-kitābay al-Mawṣūl wa-l-Ṣila*, 1–6, ed. I. ʿAbbās, M. b. Sharīfa and B. ʿAwwād Maʿrūf, Tūnis (Dār al-Gharb al-Islāmī) 2012 (Silsilat al-Tarājim al-Andalusiyya 9).

MasMur = ʿAlī ibn al-Ḥusayn al-Masʿūdī, *Murūj al-dhahab wa-maʿādin al-jawhar / Les Prairies d'Or*, 1–9, ed. and tr. C. Barbier de Meynard and [vols 1–3] P. de Courteille, Paris (Société Asiatique) 1861–1877 (Collection d'Ouvrages Orientaux).

MeGuṢa[3] = M. Meouak and P. Guichard, "al-Ṣaḳāliba", in: *EI*[2] [q.v.] s.n. (section 3).

MeGuṢM = M. Meouak and P. Guichard, "Ṣāḥib al-Madīna", in: *EI*[2] [q.v.] s.n.

MeySch = M. Meyerhof, *Über echte und unechte Schriften Galens nach arabischen Quellen*, Berlin (Verlag der Akademie der Wissenschaften) 1928 (Sitzungsberichte der Preussischen Akademie der Wissenschaften, Philologisch-Historische Klasse 28).

MoIQ = L. Molina, "Ibn al-Qūṭiyya", in: *EI*[3] [q.v.] s.n.

MPC = J. Schacht and M. Meyerhof, *The Medico-Philosophical Controversy between Ibn Butlan of Baghdad and Ibn Ridwan of Cairo. A Contribution to the History of Greek Learning among the Arabs*, Cairo (The Egyptian University) 1937 (The Faculty of Arts Publication 13).

NadFih = Muḥammad ibn Isḥāq Ibn al-Nadīm, *al-Fihrist*, 1–2, ed. G. Flügel, Leipzig (F.C.W. Vogel) 1871–1872.

NawCl = J.A. Nawas, "Client", in: *EI*[3] [q.v.] s.n.

OcJiMZ = M. Ocaña Jiménez, "Madīnat al-Zahrā'", in: *EI*[2] [q.v.] s.n.

OmFS = G. Oman, "Ricordo di Fu'ād Sayyid", in: *Oriente Moderno* 48 (1968), pp. 709–711.

OrHis = *Pauli Orosii Historiarum adversum paganos libri VII*, ed. C. Zangemeister, Lipsiae (B.G. Teubner) 1889.

OrKit = *Kitāb Hurūšiyūš (Traducción árabe de las Historiae adversus paganos de Orosio)*, ed. M. Penelas, Madrid (Consejo Superior de Investigaciones Científicas) 2001 (Fuentes Arábico-Hispanas 26).

OrTa' = *Ta'rīkh al-ʿālam: al-tarjama al-ʿarabiyya al-qadīma (muntaṣaf al-qarn al-rābiʿ al-hijrī) / Ūrūsiyūs*, ed. ʿA. al-Badawī, Bayrūt (al-Mu'assasa al-ʿArabiyya lil-Dirāsāt wa-l-Nashr) 1982.

PeJos = M. Pezeshk, "Jostanids", in: *EIr* [q.v.] s.n.

PinAM = D. Pingree, "Abū Maʿšar", in: *EIr* [q.v.] s.n.

PinTAM = D. Pingree, *The Thousands of Abū Maʿshar*, London (Warburg Institute) 1968 (Studies of the Warburg Institute 30).

PiQuo = S. Pines, "On the Pseudo-Platonic Quotation in the *Kuzari* IV and the *K. al-Nawāmīs*", in: *The Collected Works of Shlomo Pines*, vol. 5: *Studies in the History of Jewish Thought*, ed. W. Harvey, Jerusalem (Magnes Press) 1997, pp. 236–239.

PorPP = P.E. Pormann, *The Oriental Tradition of Paul of Aegina's Pragmateia*, Leiden–Boston (Brill) 2004 (Studies in Ancient Medicine 29).

PuerLP = M.J. Puertas, *Linajes y poder en la Loja islámica de los Banū Jālid a los Alatares (siglos VIII–XV)*, Motril (Fundación Ibn al-Jatib de Estudios de Cooperación Cultural) 2009.

QifTa' = ʿAlī ibn Yūsuf al-Qifṭī, *Ta'rīkh al-ḥukamā' wa-huwa mukhtaṣar al-Zawzanī al-musammā bi-l-Muntakhabāt al-multaqaṭāt min kitāb Ikhbār al-ʿulamā' bi-akhbār al-ḥukamā' li-Jamāl al-Dīn [...] al-Qifṭī*, ed. J. Lippert, Leipzig (Dieterich'sche Verlagsbuchhandlung) 1903.

ReReEn = J.C. Reeves and A.Y. Reed, *Enoch from Antiquity to the Middle Ages*, vol. 1: *Sources from Judaism, Christianity, and Islam*, Oxford (Oxford University Press) 2018.

RiUK = A. Rippin, "Ubayy b. Kaʿb", in: *EI²* [q.v.] s.n.

RMThā = R. Rashed and R. Morelon, "Th̲ābit b. Ḳurra", in: *EI²* [q.v.] s.n.

RoAC = F. Rosenthal, "An Ancient Commentary on the Hippocratic Oath", in: *Bulletin of the History of Medicine* 30 (1956), pp. 52–87.

RoHMH = F. Rosenthal, *A History of Muslim Historiography*, Leiden (E.J. Brill) 1952.

RoID = F. Rosenthal, "Ibn al-Dāya", in: *EI²* [q.v.] s.n.

RoTA = F. Rosenthal, "Isḥâq b. Ḥunayn's *Ta'rîḫ al-aṭibbâ'*", in: *Oriens* 7 (1954), pp. 55–80.

RuBīr = J. Ruska, "Al-Bīrūnī als Quelle für das Leben und die Schriften al-Rāzī's", in: *Isis* 5 (1923), pp. 26–50.

SābDis = *Sābūr ibn Sahl. The Small Dispensatory*, tr. O. Kahl, Leiden–Boston (Brill) 2003 (Islamic Philosophy, Theology and Science, Texts and Studies 53).

ṢafWā = Khalīl ibn Aybak al-Ṣafadī, *al-Wāfī bi-l-wafayāt*, 1–29, ed. A. al-Arnā'ūṭ and T. Muṣṭafā, Bayrūt (Dār Iḥyā' al-Turāth al-ʿArabī) 1420/2000.

SahOr = C.C. Sahner, "From Augustine to Islam: Translation and History in the Arabic Orosius", in: *Speculum* 88 (2013), pp. 905–931.

SánRa = I. Sánchez, "Ibn ʿAbd Rabbihi, Abū ʿUthmān", in: *EI³* [q.v.] s.n.

SaSiMC = E. de Santiago Simón, "The Itineraries of the Muslim Conquest of al-Andalus in the Light of a New Source: Ibn al-Shabbāṭ", in: *The Formation of al-Andalus. Part 1: History and Society*, ed. M. Marín, London–NewYork (Routledge) 1998 (The Formation of the Classical Islamic World 46).

ṢAṬab = Ṣāʿid ibn Aḥmad al-Andalusī, *Ṭabaqāt al-umam*, ed. L. Cheikho, Beyrouth (Imprimerie Catholique) 1912.

SchMM = W. Schmucker, *Die pflanzliche und mineralische Materia Medica im Firdaus al-Ḥikma des Ṭabarī*, Bonn (Selbstverlag des Orientalischen Seminars) 1969 (Bonner Orientalistische Studien 18).

SchUW = J. Schacht, "Umm al-Walad", in: *EI*² [q.v.] s.n.

SellIN = R. Sellheim, "Das Todesdatum des Ibn an-Nadīm", in: *Israel Oriental Studies* 2 (1972), pp. 428–432.

SellKh = R. Sellheim, "al-Khalīl b. Aḥmad", in: *EI*² [q.v.] s.n.

SellSS = J. Sellars, "Simon the Shoemaker and the Problem of Socrates", in: *Classical Philology* 98 (2003), pp. 207–216.

SezWa = U. Sezgin, "al-Waṣīfī", in: *EI*² [q.v.] s.n.

SFSS = *Seeing the Face, Seeing the Soul: Polemon's Physiognomy from Classical Antiquity to Medieval Islam*, ed. S. Swain, Oxford (Oxford University Press) 2007.

ShaGa = M. Shaki, "Gayōmart", in: *EIr* [q.v.] s.n.

SidTH = A. Sideras, "Nochmals das sogenannte *Testament des Hippokrates* (unter Berücksichtigung zweier neuer Handschriften)", in: *Sudhoffs Archiv* 90 (2006), pp. 161–202.

SkJam = P.O. Skjærvø, "Jamšid", in: *EIr* [q.v.] s.n.

SSWF = E. Savage-Smith, "The Working Files of Rhazes: Are the *Jāmiʿ* and the *Ḥāwī* identical?", in: *Medieval Arabic Thought. Essays in Honour of Fritz Zimmermann*, ed. R. Hansberger, M. Afifi al-Akiti and C. Burnett, London–Turin (Warburg Institute & Nino Aragno Editore) 2012 (Warburg Studies and Texts 4), pp. 163–180.

SSZah = E. Savage-Smith, "al-Zahrāwī", in: *EI*² [q.v.] s.n.

StDic = F. Steingass, *A Comprehensive Persian-English Dictionary*, London (Routledge & Kegan Paul) 1892.

StrḤu = G. Strohmaier, "Ḥunayn b. Isḥāq", in: *EI*³ [q.v.] s.n.

StrḤub = G. Strohmaier, "Ḥubaysh b. al-Ḥasan al-Dimashqī", in: *EI*³ [q.v.] s.n.

StrIB = G. Strohmaier, "Ibn al-Biṭrīq, Yaḥyā", in: *EI*³ [q.v.] s.n.

StrIḤ = G. Strohmaier, "Isḥāq b. Ḥunayn", in: *EI*³ [q.v.] s.n.

ṬabBP = *ʿAlī ibn Sahl Rabban aṭ-Ṭabarī's Health Regimen or "Book of the Pearl"*, ed. and tr. O. Kahl, Leiden–Boston (Brill) 2021 (Islamic Philosophy, Theology and Science, Texts and Studies 115).

ṬabIB = *ʿAlī ibn Sahl Rabban aṭ-Ṭabarī: The Indian Books*, ed. and tr. O. Kahl, Leiden–Boston (Brill) 2022 (Islamic Philosophy, Theology and Science, Texts and Studies 121).

ṬabTa' = Muḥammad ibn Jarīr al-Ṭabarī, *Ta'rīkh al-rusul wa-l-mulūk / The History of al-Ṭabarī*, vol. 23: *The Zenith of the Marwānid House*, tr. M. Hinds, Albany (State University of New York Press) 1990 (SUNY Series in Near Eastern Studies [&] Bibliotheca Persica).

TafDā = A. Tafażżoli, "Dārā(b) (1)", in: *EIr* [q.v.] s.n.

UllBei = M. Ullmann, *Beiträge zur arabischen Grammatik*, Wiesbaden (Harrassowitz) 2013.

UllFlü = M. Ullmann, *Flüche und unfromme Wünsche in der arabischen Sprache und Literatur*, Wiesbaden (Harrassowitz) 2020.

UllMed = M. Ullmann, *Die Medizin im Islam*, Leiden–Köln (E.J. Brill) 1970 (Handbuch der Orientalistik, Erste Abteilung, Der Nahe und der Mittlere Osten, Ergänzungsband 6/1).

UllMM = M. Ullmann, *Untersuchungen zur arabischen Überlieferung der Materia medica des Dioskurides. Mit Beiträgen von Rainer Degen*, Wiesbaden (Harrassowitz) 2009.

'UmMA = Aḥmad Ibn Faḍlallāh al-'Umarī, *Masālik al-abṣār fī mamālik al-amṣār*, 1–27, ed. K.S. al-Jubūrī and Mahdī al-Najm, Bayrūt (Dār al-Kutub al-'Ilmiyya) 2010.

VaIM = J.-C. Vadet, "Ibn Māsawayh", in: *EI*² [q.v.] s.n.

VerIJ = J. Vernet, "Ibn Juljul", in: *Dictionary of Scientific Biography* 7 (1973), pp. 187–188.

VerIS = J. Vernet, "Ibn Samadjūn", in: *EI*² [q.v.] s.n.

VerMA = J. Vernet, "Los médicos andaluces en el «Libro de las generaciones de médicos», de Ibn Ŷulŷul", in: *Anuario de Estudios Medievales* 5 (1968), pp. 445–462.

VerOO = J. Vernet, *Die spanisch-arabische Kultur in Orient und Okzident*, tr. K. Maier, Zürich–München (Artemis) 1984.

VuLex = I.A. Vullers, *Lexicon Persico-Latinum Etymologicum*, 1–2, Bonnae ad Rhenum (Adolph Marcus) 1855–1864.

WaḤSh = D.J. Wasserstein, "Ḥasdāy b. Shaprūṭ", in: *EI*³ [q.v.] s.n.

WgaÜ = M. Ullmann, *Wörterbuch zu den griechisch-arabischen Übersetzungen des 9. Jahrhunderts*, 1 vol. and *Supplements* 1–2, Wiesbaden (Harrassowitz) 2002 and 2006–2007.

WilJP = C. Wildberg, "John Philoponus", in: *Stanford Encyclopedia of Philosophy* [plato.stanford.edu/archives/win2021/entries/philoponus].

WisYN = R. Wisnovsky, "Yaḥyā al-Naḥwī", in: *EI*² [q.v.] s.n.

WkaS = M. Ullmann, *Wörterbuch der klassischen arabischen Sprache*, 1–2 [in 5 vols], Wiesbaden (Harrassowitz) 1970–2009.

YaBuAM = K. Yamamoto and C. Burnett, *The Great Introduction to Astrology by Abū Ma'šar*, 1–2, Leiden–Boston (Brill) 2019 (Islamic Philosophy, Theology and Science, Texts and Studies 106).

YāBul = Yāqūt ibn 'Abdallāh al-Rūmī, *Mu'jam al-buldān*, 1–10, ed. M.A. al-Khānjī, Miṣr [Cairo] (Maṭba'at al-Sa'āda) 1323/1906.

ŶulGen = *Ibn Ŷulŷul. Ṭabaqāt al-aṭibbāʾ wa-l-ḥukamāʾ "Generaciones de médicos y sabios"*, tr. E. Llavero Ruiz, Memoria de Licenciatura, Universidad de Granada, 1979 (unpublished) [downloadable at: digibug.ugr.es/handle/10481/79440].

ZakPW = M. Zakeri, *Persian Wisdom in Arabic Garb. ʿAlī b. ʿUbayda al-Rayḥānī (d. 219/834) and his Jawāhir al-kilam wa-farāʾid al-ḥikam*, 1–2, Leiden–Boston (Brill) 2007 (Islamic Philosophy, Theology and Science, Texts and Studies 66).

ZeBuMD = K.V. Zetterstéen and H. Busse, "Muʿizz al-Dawla", in: *EI*² [q.v.] s.n.

Indices

Plain numbers refer to *biographical entries* (not pages), which are counted consecutively throughout the English translation; numbers preceded by an asterisk (∗) refer to *footnotes* in this translation; numbers preceded by 'ch' refer to chapter headings (i.e. *generations*) and any uncounted material that may be attached to them; the letters P and E refer to Ibn Juljul's *Prologue* and *Epilogue*, respectively; a hyphen (-) at the beginning of a new lemma indicates the elision of the Arabic article *al*; **bold** names and numbers in index 1 ('people') signal a *main* entry in Ibn Juljul's text; lemmata that occur in a given textual entry are *not* referenced again to the footnotes which revolve around this entry. For reasons of style, terms registered in index 4 ('miscellaneous') are sometimes given as singulars *even though* they may assume a plural form in the base text.

People

Places

Work Titles

English

Arabic

Greek

Miscellaneous Terms

Arabic–English

www.ingramcontent.com/pod-product-compliance
Lightning Source LLC
Chambersburg PA
CBHW071322230926
51849CB00002B/288
* 9 7 8 9 0 0 4 6 8 2 2 2 1 *